GLUTEN-FREE
& VEGAN

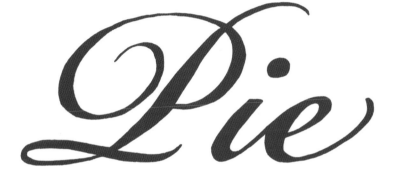

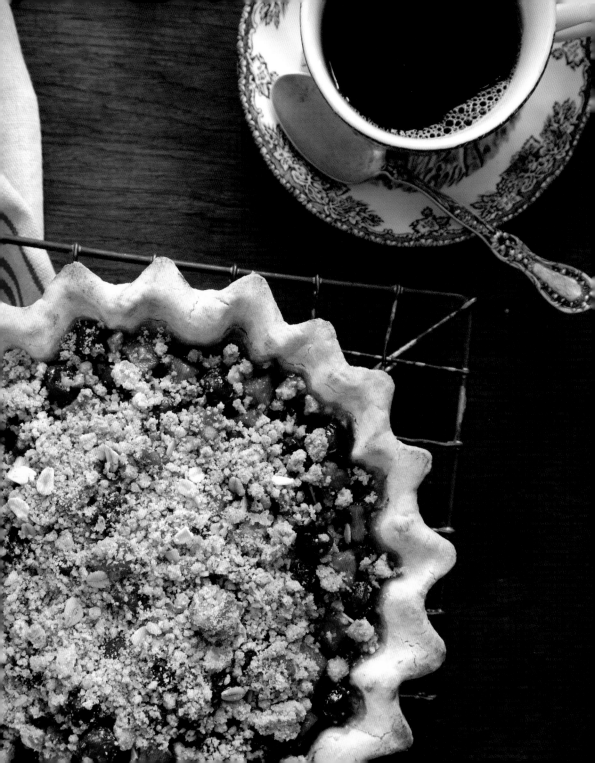

GLUTEN-FREE & VEGAN

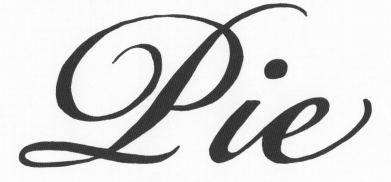

More than 50 Sweet and Savory Pies to Make at Home

JENNIFER KATZINGER

Photographs by
Charity Burggraaf

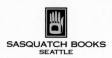

SASQUATCH BOOKS
SEATTLE

To Lilli, who believes pies are magic

✦ ✦ ✦ ✦ ✦

Printed in China

Published by Sasquatch Books
17 16 15 14 13   9 8 7 6 5 4 3 2 1

Editor: Susan Roxborough
Project editor: Michelle Hope Anderson
Design: Anna Goldstein
Photographs: Charity Burggraaf
Food styling: Julie Hopper
Copy editor: Diane Sepanski

Library of Congress Cataloging-in-Publication
Data is available.

ISBN: 978-1-57061-868-0

Sasquatch Books
1904 Third Avenue, Suite 710
Seattle, WA 98101
(206) 467-4300
www.sasquatchbooks.com
custserv@sasquatchbooks.com

CONTENTS

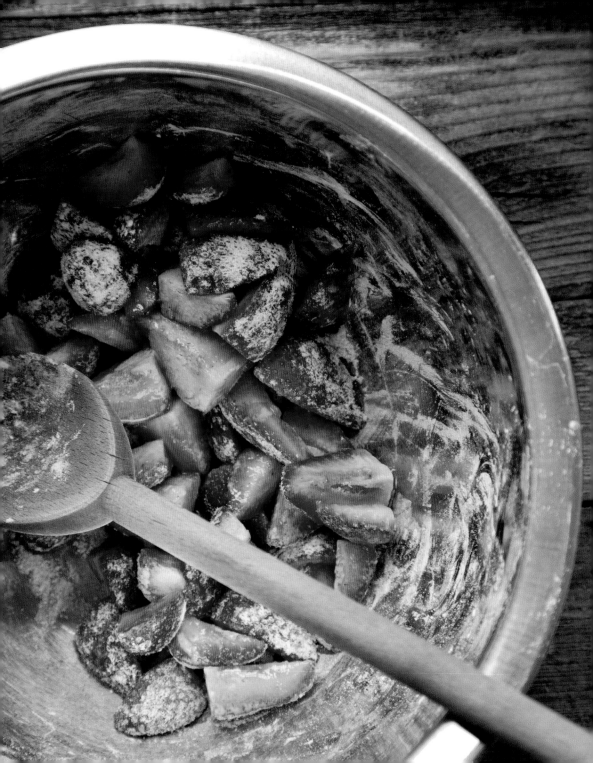

RECIPE LIST

ACKNOWLEDGMENTS

THANK YOU, JOSEPH. Your presence gives me such strength. I love you. Thank you, Lilli. Thank you for the honor and gift of being your mommy. I love you eternally. Thank you, Gabrielle, for your friendship and unobstructed beautiful energy. Thank you to all of Lilli's family. The support, joy, love, and strength you all give blossoms within her. Thank you to all of the people at Sasquatch who have put their faith in me through great times and challenging times. Thank you, Susan Roxborough, for your instructive vision and communication, and for your steady grace, poise, and positive energy. Thank you, Anna Goldstein, for your outstanding design work. Thank you, Michelle Hope Anderson, for your thorough and insightful editing. Thank you, Julie Hopper, for your exquisite food styling touch. Thank you, Charity Burggraaf, for your gorgeous photography. Thank you, Sarah Hanson, for your guidance and commitment. Thank you to the loving community I live in that surrounds me with meaningful and joyful connections.

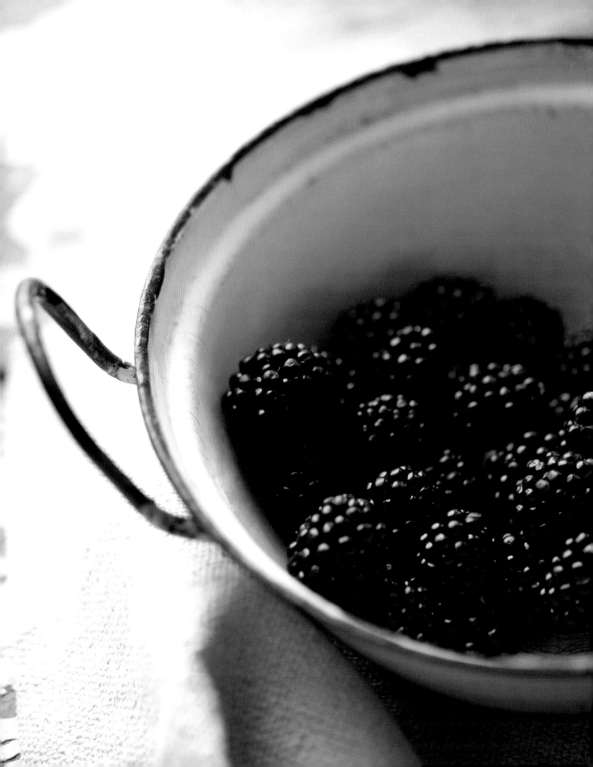

INTRODUCTION

Pie. Is there really anything else that comes close to it? If you ponder pie for just a moment, I bet nostalgic, happy, and tasty memories overcome you.

For me, writing a cookbook dedicated to pie is not only a joy, but also a great privilege. I presume that many of you interested in this book—being either gluten-free, vegan, or avoiding dairy and eggs, or a combination of these—haven't had the wonderful experience of sitting down to a piece of flaky pastry baked around a flavorful, juicy filling in quite some time. So giving you a pie you can not only eat, but also delight in, feels like a tremendous honor indeed. Pie transforms what may have been a pleasant but ordinary day into a special and festive occasion. And is it too far of a leap to suggest that the more pie you bake, the more you will gather together those dear to you?

We have an affinity for pie that surpasses any other dessert. It's not just the pie itself that captures our ardor, but the anticipation of its different varieties as the year cycles. While other desserts are perennial, pie truly expresses the changing of the seasons as we collect varying ripe fruits for luscious fillings. This cookbook is devoted to fresh, seasonal fruits—and vegetables, in the Savory Pies chapter (pages 117–135)—so I've organized most of the recipes according to the calendar's natural bounty, starting with spring and ending with winter.

Fruit and fillings aside though, I think we can all agree that a superb pie is determined by the merit of its crust. That uniquely satisfying and satiating experience of—dare I say it?—fat baked with flour into a symphony of golden delicate pastry is undoubtedly one of our tastiest treasures. That's why the most rewarding and ultimate challenge in writing this cookbook was creating the gluten-free and vegan crusts.

There are twelve crust recipes and an additional four specific to the savory pies, as well as toppings unique to the Italian Prune Plum Walnut Cobbler (page 48) and Blackberry Crumble (page 51). They vary from rolled pastry to press-in oil and nut crusts and cobbler dough. In the beginning of the crust chapters, I detail some new techniques for handling the doughs. My favorite one is what I call creating a "wedge" top crust. Basically, this is a top crust made of dough that has been rolled out into a circle and divided into eight wedges. The wedges are then placed on top of the unbaked pie, re-creating the circle. When the pie is baked, you can serve it elegantly, with ease and grace—even that usually hard-to-slice first piece!

In all my desserts, it continues to be my goal to prepare something mouthwatering and completely contenting using fewer, more healthful sweeteners. So with these recipes, I've provided just enough additional sugars to highlight the fruit and nothing more. The sweeteners vary from evaporated cane juice, brown sugar, Sucanat, molasses, and maple syrup to store-bought preserves.

There is a wide variety of pies in this book. I wanted to be sure to include a range of crusts and fillings to accommodate many desires. I'm confident you'll find just the right pie—or pies—to fulfill your cravings and create a special feast, whether it be Traditional Apple Pie (page 50), Blackberry Streusel Pie (page 42), Fresh Fruit Tart (page 75), bilberry jam–filled Linzer Torte (page 83), Pumpkin Chiffon Pie (page 113), Chocolate Prune Tart (page 82), Strawberry Hand Pies (page 93), or savory Curried Parsnip Pie (page 134)—or one of many, many more!

Many of the crusts are interchangeable; I offer recommendations in each recipe for which crusts will produce the most pleasing and delectable pie. They all have different textures and levels of sweetness. The press-in crusts are definitely more healthful than the pastry crusts, which have less fiber—but the pastry crusts are oh-so-perfect for Sweetheart Cherry Pie (page 43), Maple Blueberry Pie (page 41), and other traditional favorites!

So, dear bakers, as you delve into your precious pie-making, I congratulate you on creating some homemade magic for yourselves and those near to you!

About the
EQUIPMENT

THERE ARE A FEW KITCHEN TOOLS that will aid you greatly when making these pies.

RIMLESS BAKING SHEETS. These baking sheets are really the most beneficial when making free-form pies. Sliding your rolled-out pie dough onto a rimless baking sheet makes the process all the more graceful, but having a rimless baking sheet to slide your baked gallette off of is almost essential!

WAXED OR PARCHMENT PAPER. Please keep a roll at the ready. Either type of paper will come in handy with just about every recipe in this book. A sheet is a terrific transporter of the more fragile gluten-free dough.

9-INCH PIE PAN. All of the recipes that call for a pie pan require a 9-inch size.

SPRINGFORM PAN. Many of the cream pies are chilled in a springform pan. Removing the rim of the pan requires very little effort and makes for easy slicing and serving.

9- OR 10-INCH TART PAN WITH A REMOVABLE BOTTOM. The removable bottom makes for an elegant presentation with the side crust exposed. This also makes for easy slicing and serving.

FOOD PROCESSOR. A food processor is really essential for these recipes; it will drastically shorten the length of time it takes to make each pie dough.

ROLLING PIN. It's paramount to have a rolling pin that you are comfortable using to roll out the dough.

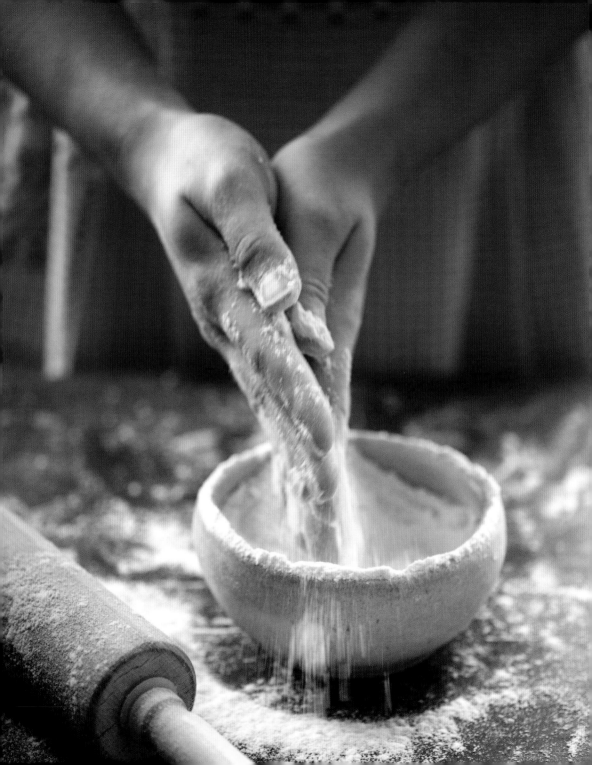

About the
INGREDIENTS

AGAR (aka agar-agar) comes from red algae. High in fiber, it's very much like gelatin in texture. It's sold powdered and in flakes; the recipes in this book call for the latter. It is used as a thickening agent.

ALMOND FLOUR, made from ground sweet almonds, has a consistency much like whole grain coarse flour. Loaded with vitamin E and magnesium, it adds a rich, nutty taste to baked goods.

ARROWROOT is unique in that it contains calcium ash and trace sea minerals. It's surprisingly unrefined: the root is simply dried and powdered. Note that it may be sold under the names arrowroot starch, arrowroot powder, and arrowroot flour—all refer to the same product.

BROWN RICE FLOUR has a very delicate flavor. It's a terrific source of fiber and contains some protein and significant amounts of the minerals selenium and magnesium. I suggest using brown rice flour to dust the work surface and rolling pin because of its mild flavor, light color, and affordability.

BROWN SUGAR is a combination of usually refined dried cane juice (white sugar) mixed with molasses. My favorite brown sugar brand is Wholesome Sweeteners.

COCONUT MILK is made from soaking grated coconut flesh in water and then extracting the liquid by mashing the softened coconut through cheesecloth. It's very high in manganese as well as iron, magnesium, phosphorus, potassium, copper, selenium, zinc, folic acid, and vitamin C. It also contains vitamin E, vitamin K, thiamin, vitamin B6, niacin, choline, pantothenic acid, and calcium.

COCONUT OIL contains lauric acid, a rare fatty acid chain that's very beneficial to our metabolism and also found in breast milk. Coconut oil is considered antiviral and antibacterial. It makes a terrific saturated fat for use in vegan pastry. Refined coconut oil has a very mild taste, while virgin coconut oil has a noticeable coconut flavor.

EVAPORATED CANE JUICE comes from sugarcane; however, it's processed to a much lesser degree than regular white sugar. Because of this, it retains more nutrients, such as riboflavin.

FLAX MEAL is very rich in omega-3 fatty acids (especially alpha-linolenic acid), lignans, and fiber. It makes an excellent substitute for eggs to bind baked goods, and also adds a small but particularly significant tasty flavor and texture. It's a wonderfully healthy food known for preventing cancers and being an anti-inflammatory.

HAZELNUTS are rich in vitamin E as well as potassium and magnesium.

MAPLE SYRUP is extracted from maple trees and then boiled to create the topping we often enjoy on pancakes. A little bit of maple syrup is a wonderful way to get the trace minerals zinc and manganese. Manganese is extremely helpful in fueling our body to create antioxidants, while zinc is a powerful mineral that fuels our immune system.

MOLASSES (BLACKSTRAP), a robust and strong sweetener, is a concentrated byproduct from making refined sugar. It's wonderfully high in iron, manganese, copper, calcium, and potassium.

OATS that are milled segregated from glutenous grains are considered gluten-free (and can be certified as such). Usually oats are milled on mills that also grind wheat, barley, rye, and the like, therefore picking up trace amounts of gluten. Thankfully, gluten-free oats are more widely available now. Oats are rich in B vitamins, iron, calcium, and vitamin E, and are very high in fiber and protein. They reduce cholesterol and regulate blood sugar, being a high-fiber food that we digest slowly.

POTATO STARCH is made by extracting the starch from potatoes. It's very mild in taste and contains high amounts of vitamin B6 and potassium, thiamine, magnesium, niacin, phosphorous, and manganese.

QUINOA FLOUR is made from ground quinoa seeds. This unique flour has a mild nutty, addictive taste. It's one of the most nutritious flours you can use, with more protein than any other flour and high in zinc, iron, calcium, vitamin B, phosphorus, potassium, magnesium, and manganese.

SORGHUM FLOUR (aka milo flour) comes from the whole grain kernel of sorghum. Nutritionally, sorghum is much like corn but higher in protein and fat. It contains many minerals such as potassium, calcium, niacin, and phosphorous. It has a very mellow taste and adds a lot of body to gluten-free breads and baked goods.

SUCANAT is a brand of whole sugarcane heated into a liquid and then cooled into crystals, thus creating a sweetener that still contains trace minerals.

TAPIOCA FLOUR is made from cassava root. The cassava root is boiled and dried, then powdered to create the flour. Tapioca contains no protein, but it does provide a little bit of folate and a fair amount of iron, as well as other minerals such as calcium, magnesium, phosphorous, potassium, zinc, copper, manganese, and selenium. I find it contributes to a very delicious golden crust and often a lighter texture, in addition to toning down the flavors of stronger-tasting flours.

TEFF FLOUR is milled from the world's smallest whole grain. Its protein content is exceptional in that it contains all eight essential amino acids and is very high in lysine, which is lacking in some plant-based foods. Teff flour is also abundant in fiber, calcium, copper, and iron, and it has a delightfully wholesome, yet subtle taste.

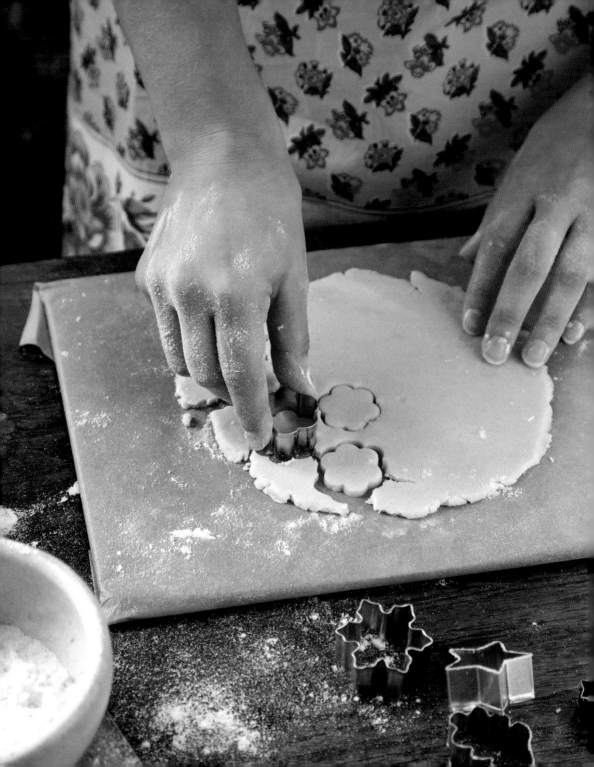

PASTRY DOUGHS

♦ ♦ ♦ ♦ ♦

♦ ♦ ♦ ♦ ♦

THE MAIN PURPOSE OF PIECRUST IS, OF COURSE, to hold your masterpiece together. Nonetheless, I'll confess that I could easily enjoy these crust recipes with or without the fillings! Before I go any further, it ought to be acknowledged that yes, gluten-free, vegan pastry is different than pastry made with butter and white wheat flour. As the saying goes, they are apples and oranges. However, I am confident that you'll agree these crusts are absolutely heavenly as they melt in your mouth, utterly tender, and provide an amazing vehicle for fruit, cream, nut, and chocolate fillings.

Pastry Dough Tips and Techniques

MAKING A CRUST THAT REPEATEDLY MEETS your highest expectations time and time again is quite challenging. Many factors are at play that influence the outcome of your pastry, such as the temperature of the ingredients and how the flours are measured. I give detailed instructions in each recipe that I believe you'll find very helpful in creating a reliable and excellent crust, but before jumping in, please read these extra tips.

MEASURING FLOUR: When it comes to measuring flour, it is preferable to scoop it into your measuring cup, slightly overfilling it. Next, use a butter knife to scrape the excess off the top of the cup before using the flour in your recipe.

MEASURING AND STORING COCONUT OIL: I recommend storing coconut oil in the cupboard, as it's much easier to scoop at room temperature.

COMBINING FLOUR AND COCONUT OIL: Mix the coconut oil and flour until you have little balls that are about the size of a pebble, or about half the size of a pea. Then add the water and vanilla extract, and mix until your dough holds together. This may take up to two or three minutes.

ROLLING OUT THE BOTTOM CRUST: Once your dough is ready, generously flour your work surface with brown rice flour and use your hands to pat the dough into a circle. Dust both your rolling pin and the disc with brown rice flour. Following are two ways to roll out the dough. Whichever method you choose, remember the circle doesn't have to be perfect, as you will smooth the edges when you flute or crimp them (see "Fluting the bottom crust," page 5).

1. The simpler way is just to roll out the disc on a large, well-floured piece of parchment paper. Using parchment paper makes it convenient to rotate the dough as you roll it, which ensures a more uniform circular shape to fit your pan (rather than an oblong shape). It also helps you transfer the dough to a pie or tart pan or, for the free-form hand pies, onto a baking sheet.

2. You can also purchase a strong piece of cardboard or a very thin cutting board (such as bamboo), measuring at least 12 by 12 inches. You can pick up a sheet cake board cheaply at your local bakery and cut it down to size with an X-ACTO knife. Tape your parchment paper to the board, folding it over so the tape is on the back. Then each time you use the board, you can change the parchment. Just flour it and roll out your pastry. The cake board will last indefinitely for countless piecrusts and is also helpful when it comes time to flip the rolled-out dough into the pie pan.

FLIPPING THE ROLLED-OUT BOTTOM CRUST INTO THE PAN:

1. If you rolled the dough out on parchment paper, simply slide the palm of your hand underneath the dough on the parchment and flip it into your pie pan. Gently peel back the paper and proceed to fit your pie. This may result in some tears in the pastry (see "Repairing tears in the dough," following).

2. If you rolled the dough out on the lined cake board, position the pie pan or tart pan so it is directly centered on top of the dough face-down. With one

hand underneath the board and one hand on the bottom of the plate, flip the two together so the pie pan is positioned upright with the cake board above. Remove the board and parchment, and press the dough into the pan. You will most likely have some tears in the pastry: in fact, expect them (see "Repairing tears in the dough," below).

REPAIRING TEARS IN THE DOUGH: Gluten-free pastry doesn't have the elasticity of conventional pastry dough and, as a result, is more fragile. Not to worry though! Tears can easily be mended: simply dust clean hands in brown rice flour and press the dough back together. I also designed the double-crust recipes to allow for extra dough, so when a tear occurs on a rolled-out upper crust (for example, during the transfer to the pie pan or as the dough stretches over the bumpy fruit filling), you can roll out the extra dough and cut it into decorative leaves, hearts, or other shapes, then place them gracefully over the tear, making for an adorable pie.

FLUTING THE BOTTOM CRUST AND FITTING THE PAN: I like to create a thicker side wall for a sturdy and defined flute on my pies, as well as a thinner bottom crust. To do this, make sure your hands are clean, dry, and dusted with brown rice flour. With the palm of whichever hand you predominately use, press against the bottom crust in a circular pattern while your other hand rotates the pie pan. This will push the dough up the sides of your pie pan while creating a lighter bottom crust. Then, to finish off the sides, fold the dough under, or press and squeeze it evenly into the top edge of the pan.

To flute the pastry for a single crust, pinch the dough between your thumb and index finger. Begin by resting the thumb and index finger of whichever hand you predominantly use on a spot on the crust's edge, with the tip of your thumb and finger on the inside perimeter. Place your index finger in between your nondominant thumb and other index finger on the outside of the pie perimeter. Now pull the dough by moving your nondominant index finger toward the center of the pie about ¼ inch as your thumb and other index finger simultaneously pull the dough toward the outside of the pie ¼ inch.

A simpler but also delightful design to finish the edge is to use a floured fork and press the dough down gently to form a pattern with the tines. A spoon pressed facedown to create a V-like shape is also a very cute option.

All but two of my double-crust pies have a wedge or cutout top crust. Simply flute the bottom crust as described on page 5, just as you would for a single-crust or streusel-topped pie, and proceed to make top crust as described below.

ROLLING OUT THE TOP CRUST: There are only two recipes in which I call for a traditional top crust that covers the whole pie (and for those, I give instructions on how to roll out the top crust within the recipe). For the rest of the double-crust recipes, I use either a wedge top crust or a top crust with hearts or other cutouts:

MAKING A WEDGE TOP CRUST: For many recipes, I like to make eight wedges that fit together smoothly and attractively over the filling. To create the wedges, you will need a 9-inch removable tart pan bottom as a template. Generously flour it, then roll out your top crust on top of it to about an ⅛-inch thickness. Trim off the excess dough so that you have a perfect circle. With a sharp knife, cut the circle into eight equal wedges. Use a knife or a spatula to slightly and gently separate the wedges and then transfer to a parchment-lined flat surface to prevent them from sticking together when you freeze the dough. Place the wedges in the freezer, uncovered, for 30 minutes.

For a fun and fancy appearance, you can also use a small, well-floured cookie cutter (circle, star, leaf, etc.) to cut and remove a decorative shape from each wedge to show a little of the filling.

MAKING A TOP CRUST WITH HEARTS OR OTHER CUTOUTS: In some recipes, I call for hearts or other cutout shapes. For these, simply roll out the dough to approximately ⅛-inch thickness and cut out varying sizes of hearts. Use a spatula to transfer them to a baking sheet well dusted with flour and freeze them for approximately 30 minutes, or until stiff. Place the larger ones close to the edge of the pie and the smaller ones toward the middle. You can also alternate the direction of the cutouts; this will allow you to fit more on top.

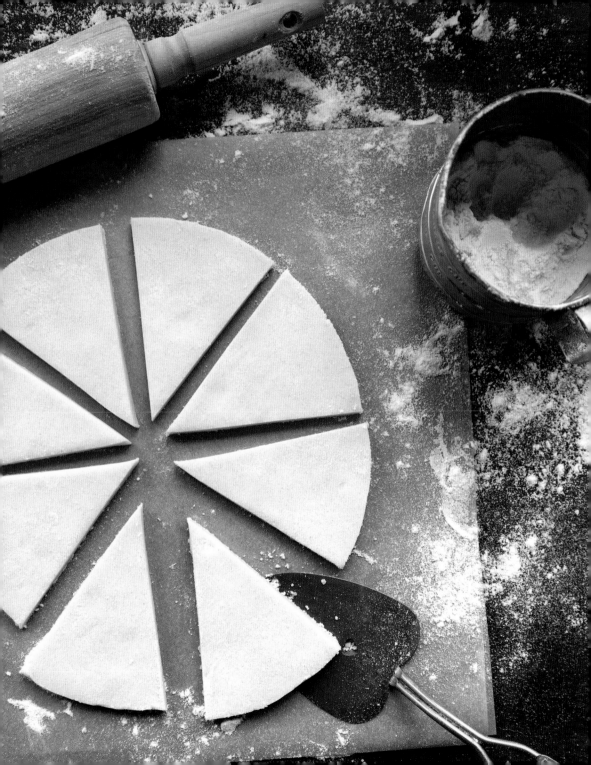

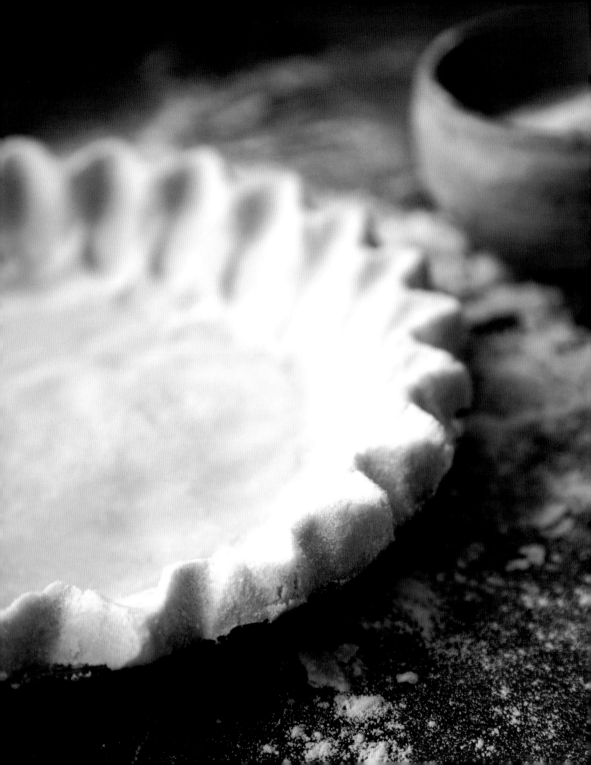

⬩ Single Pastry Crust ⬩

This is basically the same dough as for the Double Pastry Crust (page 11), but the instructions and techniques for handling the doughs vary, which is why I've separated the recipes. This particular single pastry is terrific for making tarts and free-form pies. I also recommend this crust for the cream pies.

〰〰〰〰〰〰〰〰〰〰〰〰〰〰〰 **MAKES 1 SINGLE CRUST** 〰〰〰〰〰〰〰〰〰〰〰〰〰〰〰

1 cup brown rice flour

3 tablespoons tapioca flour

⅓ cup potato starch

2½ tablespoons arrowroot

2½ teaspoons evaporated cane juice

¼ teaspoon salt

¼ teaspoon lemon zest

½ cup plus 1 tablespoon refined coconut oil

2 tablespoons water

1 teaspoon vanilla extract

1. Place the flours, potato starch, arrowroot, evaporated cane juice, salt, and lemon zest in the bowl of a food processor and process just until the ingredients are combined. Add the coconut oil and pulse until the dough is the consistency of coarse meal with many pebble-size pieces. Add the water and vanilla, and process until the dough holds together.

> **NOTE:** For the Free-Form Pies (pages 55–69), you will prepare the crust up until this point only. Proceed to your specific recipe for instructions on how to roll out, fill, and bake the crust.
>
> The directions that follow apply if you're making a cream pie or tart. Check your recipe to see what specific pan is called for before you proceed with this step.

2. Place the dough on a piece of parchment paper well dusted with brown rice flour. Shape it into a disc with your hands. Dust both your rolling pin and the disc with brown rice flour. As you roll out the dough, rotate the paper so you roll in different directions to produce an 11-inch circle.

continued

3. Working quickly, slip your hand under the parchment paper to lift up the dough and flip it into the pie pan. Or if you're making a tart, slide the removable tart bottom underneath the dough, lifting it off the parchment, then set the bottom into the pan's fluted rim. Using the palm of your dominant hand, press evenly and gently into the dough at the base of the pan while rotating the pan every so often. This will create a thinner bottom crust and thicker side walls. Then press the extra dough into the rim with your fingertips to shape the edges uniformly.

4. For pies, flute or decoratively crimp the edges of the dough, (see "Fluting the bottom crust," page 5).

5. Pierce the dough all over with a fork to prevent air pockets from forming when baking, and freeze it, uncovered, for 30 to 45 minutes before filling.

NOTE: At this point, proceed to your recipe for instructions on how to fill and bake the crust.

✦ Double Pastry Crust ✦

This rich dough is reminiscent of a tender shortbread. It melts in your mouth and is just sweet enough to subtly accent the pie filling. The texture is flaky yet sufficiently robust to hold ample fruit, cream, or chocolate fillings.

|||||||||||||||||||||||||||||||||||||||| **MAKES 1 DOUBLE CRUST** ||||||||||||||||||||||||||||||||||||||||

2 cups brown rice flour

⅓ cup tapioca flour

⅔ cup potato starch

⅓ cup arrowroot

1½ tablespoons evaporated cane juice

¾ teaspoon salt

½ teaspoon lemon zest

1 cup plus 2 tablespoons refined coconut oil

2 tablespoons water

2 teaspoons vanilla extract

||||||||||||||||||||||||||||||||||||||||||||||||||||||||||||||||||||||||||||||||||||||||||||||||||||||||||||||||||||||||||||||||||||||||||

1. Place the flours, potato starch, arrowroot, evaporated cane juice, salt, and lemon zest in the bowl of a food processor and process just until the ingredients are combined. Add the coconut oil and pulse until the dough is the consistency of coarse meal with many pearl-size pieces. Add the water and vanilla, and process just until the dough holds together.

> **NOTE:** For the Plum Galette (page 63), you will prepare the dough up until this point only. Proceed to the recipe for instructions on how to roll out, fill, and bake the crust.
>
> The directions that follow apply if you're making a sweet pie. Check your recipe to see what specific pan is called for before you proceed with this step.

2. Place the dough on a piece of parchment paper well dusted with brown rice flour. Divide it into two portions, one slightly larger (about two-thirds of the dough) than the other; this will be the bottom crust. Shape the larger portion into a disc with your hands. Dust both your rolling pin and the disc with brown rice flour. As you roll out the dough, rotate the paper so you roll in different directions to produce an 11-inch circle.

continued

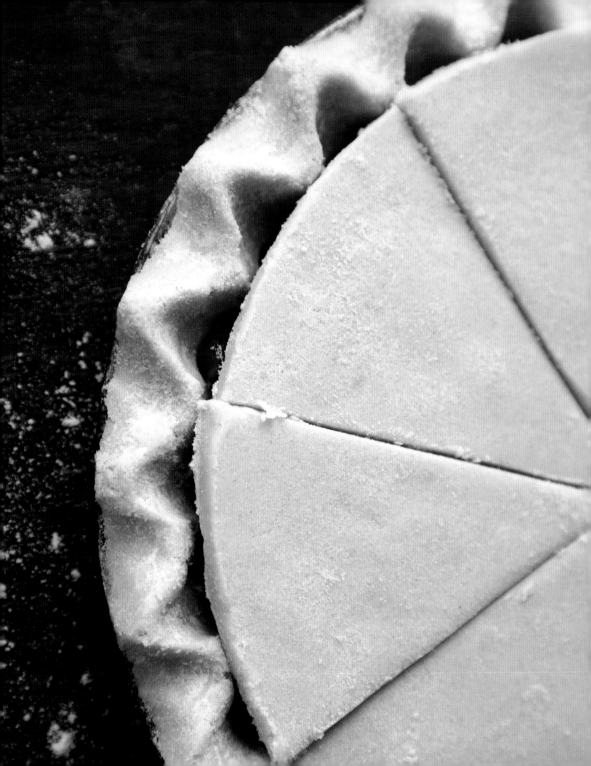

3. Working quickly, slip your hand under the parchment paper to lift up the dough and flip it into the pie pan. Using the palm of your dominant hand, press evenly and gently into the dough at the base of the pan while rotating the pan every so often. This will create a thinner bottom crust and thicker side walls. Then press the extra dough into the rim with your fingertips to shape the edges uniformly.

4. Flute or decoratively crimp the edges of the dough (see "Fluting the bottom crust," page 5). Pierce the dough all over with a fork to prevent air pockets from forming when baking, uncovered, and freeze it for 30 to 45 minutes before filling.

> NOTE: Two of the double-crust recipes in this book, Traditional Apple Pie (page 50) and Summer Peach Pie (page 45), call for a traditional top crust—a large piece of pastry that completely covers the filling. For those, make the bottom crust up until this point, then proceed to the recipes for instructions on how to make the top crust.

5. Roll out the remaining portion of dough to about ⅛-inch thickness to create the top crust, either cutting out hearts or other shapes, or creating wedges by rolling out the dough on the bottom of a 9-inch tart pan, trimming it to fit, and cutting it into wedges (see "Making a top crust with hearts or other cutouts" or "Making a wedge top crust," page 6). Freeze the cutouts or wedges for 30 minutes.

6. After the dough has been frozen, remove it from the freezer and fill the bottom crust according to your specific recipe. To assemble the top crust, gently loosen the wedges from the parchment with a spatula and place each wedge next to one another, re-creating your circle. If you're using cutouts, proceed in the same manner.

> NOTE: At this point, proceed to your recipe for instructions on how to fill and bake the crust.

◆ Darker Double Crust ◆

The dough in this recipe is darker due to the addition of teff flour, which also lends a wholesome and slightly heartier texture to the pastry in a delicious and subtle manner. Use this in any of the pie recipes that call for a double crust. You may want to experiment with both the lighter and darker crusts to see which one you prefer with which fillings.

IIIIIIIIIIIIIIIIIIIIIIIIIIIIIIIIIIIIIIIII **MAKES 1 DOUBLE CRUST** IIIIIIIIIIIIIIIIIIIIIIIIIIIIIIIIIIIIIIIIIIII

1½ cups brown rice flour

½ cup teff flour

⅓ cup tapioca flour

⅔ cup potato starch

⅓ cup arrowroot

1½ tablespoons evaporated cane juice

¾ teaspoon salt

½ teaspoon lemon zest

1 cup plus 2 tablespoons refined coconut oil

3 tablespoons water

2 teaspoons vanilla extract

IIIIIIIIIIIIIIIIIIIIIIIIIIIIIIIIIIIIIIIIIIIIIIIIIIIIIIIIIIIIIIIIIIIIIIIIIIIIIIIIIIIIIIIIIIIIIIIIIIIIIIIIIIIIIIIIIIIIIIIIIIIIIIIIIIIIIIIIIIIIIIIII

1. Place the flours, potato starch, arrowroot, evaporated cane juice, salt, and lemon zest in the bowl of a food processor and process just until the ingredients are combined. Add the coconut oil and pulse until the dough is the consistency of coarse meal with many pearl-size pieces. Add the water and vanilla, and process just until the dough holds together.

    NOTE: For the Plum Galette (page 63), you will prepare the dough up until this point only. Proceed to the recipe for instructions on how to roll out, fill, and bake the crust.

    The directions that follow apply if you're making a sweet pie. Check your recipe to see what specific pan is called for before you proceed with this step.

2. Place the dough on a piece of parchment paper well dusted with brown rice flour. Divide it into two portions, one slightly larger (about two-thirds of the dough) than the other; this will be the bottom crust. Shape the larger portion into a disc with your hands. Dust both your rolling pin and the disc with brown rice flour. As you

roll out the dough, rotate the paper so you roll in different directions to produce an 11-inch circle.

3. Working quickly, slip your hand under the parchment paper to lift up the dough and flip it into the pie pan. Using the palm of your dominant hand, press evenly and gently into the dough at the base of the pan while rotating the pan every so often. This will create a thinner bottom crust and thicker side walls. Then press the extra dough into the rim with your fingertips to shape the edges uniformly.

4. Flute or decoratively crimp the edges of the dough (see "Fluting the bottom crust," page 5). Pierce the dough all over with a fork to prevent air pockets from forming when baking, and freeze it, uncovered, for 45 minutes before filling.

> NOTE: Two of the double-crust recipes in this book, Traditional Apple Pie (page 50) and Summer Peach Pie (page 45), call for a traditional top crust—a large piece of pastry that completely covers the filling. For those, make the bottom crust up until this point, then proceed to the recipes for instructions on how to make the top crust.

5. Roll out the remaining portion of dough to about ⅛-inch thickness to create the top crust, either cutting out hearts or other shapes, or creating wedges by rolling out the dough on the bottom of a 9-inch tart pan, trimming it to fit, and cutting it into wedges (see "Making a top crust with hearts or other cutouts" or "Making a wedge top crust," page 6). Freeze the cutouts or wedges for 30 minutes.

6. After the dough has been frozen, remove it from the freezer and fill the bottom crust according your specific recipe. To assemble the top crust, gently loosen the wedges from the parchment with a spatula and place each wedge next to one another, re-creating your circle. If you're using cutouts, proceed in the same manner.

> NOTE: At this point, proceed to your recipe for instructions on how to fill and bake the crust.

⬩ Single Crust with Streusel Topping ⬩

A streusel topping is uniquely wonderful with its nutty, crunchy, cinnamony bursts. It's also super easy to assemble. If you're shy on time or prefer this style and taste of pie, you can substitute this crust for any of the fruit pies that call for a Double Pastry Crust or Darker Double Crust.

||||||||||||||||||||||||||||||||||||||||||||||| **MAKES 1 CRUST** |||||||||||||||||||||||||||||||||||||||||||||||||

2 cups brown rice flour

⅓ cup tapioca flour

⅔ cup potato starch

⅓ cup arrowroot

1½ tablespoons evaporated cane juice

¾ teaspoon salt

1 cup plus 2 tablespoons refined coconut oil

2 tablespoons water

2 teaspoons vanilla extract

¾ cup gluten-free oats

½ cup chopped pecans or walnuts

2½ tablespoons maple syrup

1 teaspoon ground cinnamon

|||||||||||||||||||||||||||||||||||||||||||||||||||||||||||||||||||||||||||||||||||||||||||||||||||||||||||||||||||||||||

1. Place the flours, potato starch, arrowroot, evaporated cane juice, and salt in the bowl of a food processor and process just until the ingredients are combined. Add the coconut oil and pulse until the dough is the consistency of coarse meal with many pearl-size dough pieces. Add the water and vanilla and process until the dough holds together.

2. Place the dough on a piece of parchment paper well dusted with brown rice flour. Divide it into two portions, one slightly larger (about ⅔ of the dough) than the other: this will be the bottom crust. (You'll use the smaller portion to create the streusel topping.) Shape the larger portion into a disc with your hands. Dust both your rolling pin and the disc with brown rice flour. As you roll out the dough, rotate the paper so you roll in different directions to produce a 11-inch circle.

3. Working quickly, slip your hand under the parchment paper to lift up the dough and flip it into the pie pan. Using the palm of your hand, press evenly and gently into the dough that is resting on the base of the pan while rotating the pan every so often. This will create a thinner bottom crust and thicker side walls. Go ahead and use

your hands around the perimeter to shape the edges uniformly, pressing into the rim the extra dough that rose up the sides as you created your thinner bottom crust.

4. Flute or decoratively crimp the edges of the dough (see "Fluting the bottom crust," page 5). Pierce the dough all over with a fork and freeze it for 45 minutes before filling.

5. To make the streusel topping, place the remaining ⅓ portion of dough into a food processor with the oats, pecans, maple syrup, and cinnamon. Pulse until mixture is crumbly, but some of the nuts are still intact. After you fill the pie, sprinkle the streusel evenly over the top and bake per recipe instructions.

NOTE: At this point, proceed to your recipe for instructions on how to fill and bake the crust.

✦ Hazelnut Pastry Crust ✦

I really enjoy working with this very smooth dough. A generous quantity of finely ground toasted hazelnuts gives it a rich nutty flavor and earthy sweetness.

||||||||||||||||||||||||||||||||||||||||||| **MAKES 1 DOUBLE CRUST** |||||||||||||||||||||||||||||||||||||||||||

1 cup hazelnuts

1¾ cups brown rice flour

⅓ cup tapioca flour

⅓ cup potato starch

⅓ cup arrowroot

1½ tablespoons evaporated cane juice

½ teaspoon baking powder

1 teaspoon ground cinnamon

¾ teaspoon salt

1 cup refined coconut oil

2 tablespoons water

2 teaspoons vanilla extract

|||||||||||||||||||||||||||||||||||||||||||||||||||||||||||||||||||||||||||||||||||||||||||||||||||||||||||||||||||||

1. Preheat the oven to 350 degrees F. Spread the hazelnuts out on a baking sheet in one layer. When the oven is hot, toast the hazelnuts for about 12 minutes, or until they are lightly browned, fragrant, and the skins blistered. Rub the hazelnuts in a clean kitchen towel to remove their skins (some skins will not come off; don't worry about those). Cool the hazelnuts completely and then grind in the bowl of a food processor—pulse just a few times or you will end up with nut butter. You should end up with about ¾ cup of ground hazelnuts.

2. Place the ground hazelnuts, flours, potato starch, arrowroot, evaporated cane juice, baking powder, cinnamon, and salt in the cleaned food processor bowl and process just until the ingredients are combined.

3. Add the coconut oil and pulse until the dough is the consistency of coarse meal with many pearl-size dough pieces. Add the water and vanilla and process until the dough holds together.

NOTE: For the Linzer Torte (page 83), you will prepare the dough up until this point only. Proceed to the recipe for instructions on how to roll out, fill, and bake the crust.

4. Divide the dough into two portions, one portion will be slightly larger for your bottom crust. Place the large portion of the dough on a piece of parchment paper well dusted with brown rice flour. Shape it into a disc with your hands. Dust both your rolling pin and the disc with brown rice flour. As you roll out the dough, rotate the paper so you roll in different directions to produce a 11-inch circle.

5. Working quickly, slip your hand under the parchment paper to lift up the dough and flip it into the pie pan.

6. Flute or decoratively crimp the edges of the dough (see "Fluting the bottom crust," page 5). Pierce the dough all over with a fork and freeze it for 45 minutes before filling.

7. Roll out the remaining portion of dough to about ⅛-inch thickness to create the top crust, either cutting out hearts or leaf shapes. Transfer the cutouts with the aid of a spatula to a generously floured surface. Place in the freezer for about 30 minutes to harden before assembling your pie.

NOTE: At this point, proceed to your recipe for instructions on how to fill and bake the crust.

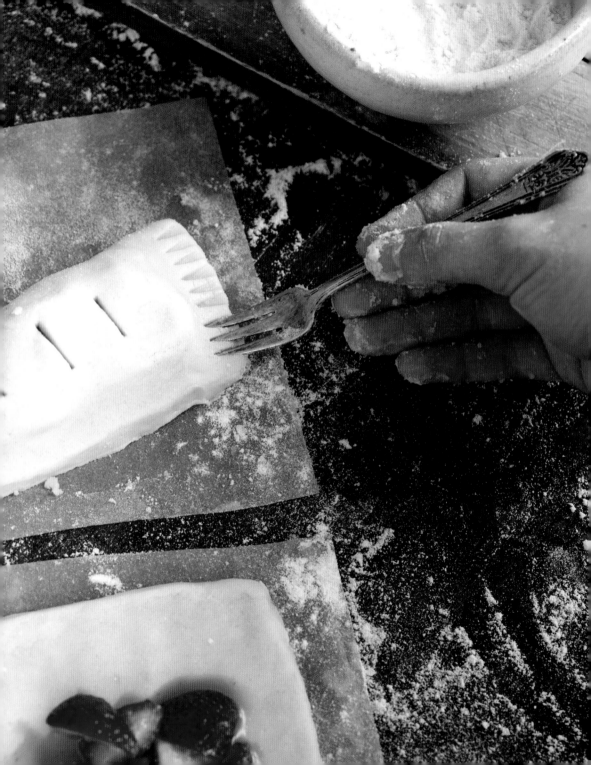

✦ Hand Pie and Turnover Dough ✦

This dough differs from the Single and Double Pastry Crust doughs in its slightly increased amount of coconut oil. The extra oil makes for a more supple dough that is easier to handle. It also enhances the flakiness of the hand pie, creating a texture akin to a turnover.

‖‖‖‖‖‖‖‖‖‖‖‖‖‖‖‖‖‖‖‖‖‖‖‖‖‖‖‖‖‖‖‖‖ **MAKES 8 HAND PIES** ‖‖‖‖‖‖‖‖‖‖‖‖‖‖‖‖‖‖‖‖‖‖‖‖‖‖‖‖‖‖‖‖‖

2 cups brown rice flour

⅓ cup tapioca flour

1 cup potato starch

1 tablespoon evaporated cane juice

½ teaspoon salt

1 cup plus 2 tablespoons refined coconut oil

2 teaspoons vanilla extract

2 tablespoons plus 2 teaspoons water

‖‖‖

1. Place the flours, potato starch, evaporated cane juice, and salt in the bowl of a food processor and process just until the ingredients are combined. Add the coconut oil and pulse until the dough is the consistency of coarse meal with many pearl-size dough pieces. Add the water and vanilla, and process until the dough holds together.

   NOTE: At this point, proceed to your recipe for instructions on how to roll and shape the dough and fill and bake the crust.

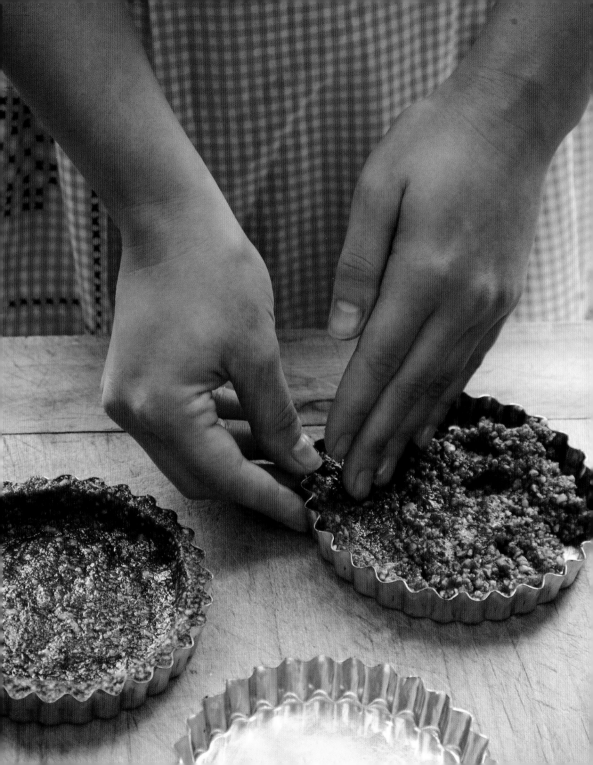

PRESS-IN CRUSTS

✦ ✦ ✦ ✦ ✦

✦ ✦ ✦ ✦ ✦

T HESE PRESS-IN CRUSTS ARE DISTINCTIVE IN TASTE and structure, reminding me of daintily sweetened "buttery" shortbreads, abundant with almonds, pecans, and walnuts. Surprisingly, while they're so rich in character, they actually come together with very little effort. I enjoy pressing the tender doughs into their pans—there's something rather liberating about making a piecrust sans the rolling pin!

PRESS-IN CRUST TIP AND TECHNIQUE

HOW TO PROCESS THE NUTS: Process the nuts until they are finely ground but not so much that they turn into nut butter. To do this, pulse your food processor rather than let it process continuously. You will have more control this way.

✦ Almond Press-In Crust ✦

This crust has a subtly sweet almond flavor and a cookielike texture. It's a crisp and nutty complement to a fruit or cream filling. It makes for a mellow backdrop and accentuates the filling of your pie.

IIIIIIIIIIIIIIIIIIIIIIIIIIIIIIIIIIIIIIIIIIIIIIIIIII **MAKES 1 CRUST** IIIIIIIIIIIIIIIIIIIIIIIIIIIIIIIIIIIIIIIIIIIIIIIIIII

2 cups almond flour

2 tablespoons coconut oil

2 tablespoons maple syrup

1 teaspoon vanilla extract

Pinch of salt

IIIIIIIIIIIIIIIIIIIIIIIIIIIIIIIIIIIIIIIIIIIIIIIIIIIIIIIIIIIIIIIIIIIIIIIIIIIIIIIIIIIIIIIIIIIIIIIIIIIIIIIIIIIIIIIIIIIIIII

1. Preheat the oven to 350 degrees F.

2. Place all the ingredients in the bowl of a food processor and mix just until the dough resembles fine meal. Do not overprocess. The dough will be sticky.

3. With clean, damp hands, press the dough into the pan called for in the recipe you're making.

4. Bake, uncovered, for 15 minutes, or until the crust smells like toasted almonds. It will be golden and firm to the touch. Let it cool completely before filling, about 1½ hours.

✦ Chocolate Almond Press-In Crust ✦

Yes, I do love chocolate—if you haven't noticed already, there are two chocolate press-in crust recipes in this book. However, the Dark Chocolate Pecan Press-In Crust (page 30) has a distinctive pecan richness, while this recipe, made with almond flour, has a different texture and, of course, taste. Each being so delicious, I just had to include both.

||||||||||||||||||||||||||||||||||||||||||||| **MAKES 1 CRUST** |||||||||||||||||||||||||||||||||||||||||||||

1¾ cups almond flour

½ cup cocoa powder

2½ tablespoons coconut oil

2 tablespoons maple syrup

1 teaspoon vanilla extract

Pinch of salt

|||||||||||||||||||||||||||||||||||||||||||||||||||||||||||||||||||||||||||||||||||||||||||||||||||||||||||||||||||||||||||

1. Preheat the oven to 350 degrees F.

2. Place all the ingredients in the bowl of a food processor and mix just until the dough resembles fine meal. Do not overprocess. The dough will be sticky.

3. With clean, damp hands, press the dough into the pan called for in the recipe you're making.

4. Bake, uncovered, for 15 minutes until the crust smells like just-baked cookies. It will be slightly darker and firm to the touch. Let it cool completely before filling, about 1½ hours.

✦ Ginger Pecan Press-In Crust ✦

This crust awakens the palate with delightful bursts of warming spices and a bit of sweetening from molasses and maple syrup. The ground pecans caramelize and deepen in flavor as they bake into a heavenly base for your pie or tart. This crust is spectacular with the Fresh Fruit Tart (page 75), and most of the Cream Pies (page 103)—especially the Chocolate Cream Pie (page 114).

|||||||||||||||||||||||||||||||||||||||||||||||||| **MAKES 1 CRUST** ||||||||||||||||||||||||||||||||||||||||||||||||||

1½ cups ground pecans

2 tablespoons canola oil

1 tablespoon maple syrup

1 tablespoon blackstrap molasses

¾ teaspoon peeled and grated
    fresh ginger

1 teaspoon ground cinnamon

¼ teaspoon ground cloves

1 teaspoon vanilla extract

Pinch of salt

1. Preheat the oven to 350 degrees F.

2. Place all the ingredients in the bowl of a food processor and mix just until the dough holds together. Do not overprocess. The dough will be sticky.

3. With clean, damp hands, press the dough into the pan called for in the recipe you're making. Bake, uncovered, for 15 minutes, or until the crust smells like toasted pecans. It will be slightly darker and firm to the touch. Let it cool completely before filling, about 1½ hours.

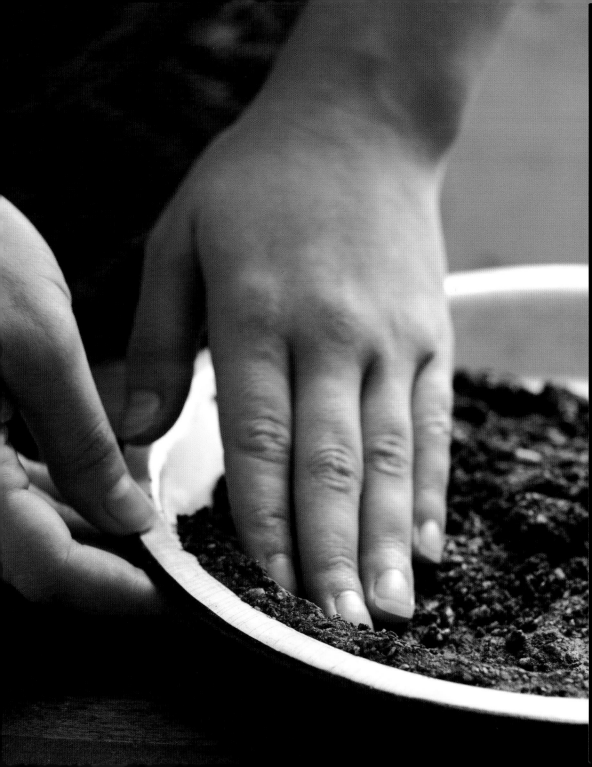

◆ Dark Chocolate Pecan Press-In Crust ◆

Rich with chocolate, this crust is so tasty, it could satisfy even without a filling. As the backdrop of your tart or cream pie, the crust influences the experience of deliciousness. In the case of this crust, the chocolate interacts with your filling in a complex and satisfying way. This crust has more of an impact than non-chocolate press-in crusts. I recommend this crust with any of the chocolate pies, as well as the Grasshopper Pie (page 109) and the Pumpkin Chiffon Pie (page 113).

MAKES 1 CRUST

1½ cups ground pecans

½ cup cocoa powder

2 tablespoons canola oil

2 tablespoons maple syrup

1 teaspoon vanilla extract

Pinch of salt

1. Preheat the oven to 350 degrees F.

2. Place all the ingredients in the bowl of a food processor and mix just until the dough resembles fine meal. Do not overprocess. The dough will be sticky.

3. With clean, damp hands, press the dough into the pan called for in the recipe you're making.

4. Bake, uncovered, for 20 minutes, or until the crust smells like just-baked cookies. It will be slightly darker and firm to the touch. Let it cool completely before filling, about 1½ hours.

✦ Olive Oil Press-In Crust ✦

Oil crusts are very tasty and unique. They make especially terrific single crusts for pies and especially tarts. This particular crust has a delicately sweet and nutty taste. The Italians know how amazing olive oil is in baked goods—it's also exceptional in a tender pastry crust.

||||||||||||||||||||||||||||||||||||||||||||||||| **MAKES 1 CRUST** |||||||||||||||||||||||||||||||||||||||||||||||||

2 cups brown rice flour	1 tablespoon evaporated cane juice
⅓ cup potato starch	¼ teaspoon salt
⅓ cup tapioca flour	½ cup plus 2 tablespoons olive oil

|||||||||||||||||||||||||||||||||||||||||||||||||||||||||||||||||||||||||||||||||||||||||||||||||||||||||||||||||||||||||||||||

1. Preheat the oven to 350 degrees F.

2. Place all the ingredients in the bowl of a food processor and mix just until the dough becomes soft. Do not overprocess. The dough will be sticky.

3. With clean, damp hands, press the dough into the pan called for in the recipe you're making.

4. Pierce it all over with a fork and place the pan, uncovered, in the freezer for 45 minutes prior to baking.

5. Remove the pan from the freezer and bake for 35 minutes, or until the crust is golden and firm to the touch. Let it cool for 1 hour before filling.

✦ Canola Oil Walnut Press-In Crust ✦

This is a handy recipe should you ever long to make a tart and are out of coconut oil. It's nice to have an option for making a dough with different oils, whether saturated or unsaturated. With toasted walnuts and a hint of cinnamon, this crust is most satisfying for the taste buds.

||||||||||||||||||||||||||||||||||||||||||||||||||||| **MAKES 1 CRUST** |||||||||||||||||||||||||||||||||||||||||||||||||||||

½ cup toasted walnuts

1 cup brown rice flour

⅓ cup sweet white sorghum flour

¼ cup tapioca flour

½ teaspoon salt

1 tablespoon Sucanat

½ teaspoon cinnamon

½ cup canola oil

|||||||||||||||||||||||||||||||||||||||||||||||||||||||||||||||||||||||||||||||||||||||||||||||||||||||||||||||||||||||||||||

1. Preheat the oven to 350 degrees F.

2. Place all the ingredients in the bowl of a food processor and mix just until the dough becomes soft. Do not overprocess. The dough will be sticky.

3. With clean, damp hands, press the dough into the pan called for in the recipe you're making.

4. Pierce it all over with a fork and place the pan, uncovered, in the freezer for 45 minutes prior to baking.

5. Remove the pan from the freezer and bake the crust for 25 minutes, or until it smells like toasted walnuts. It will be golden and firm to the touch. Let it cool for 1 hour before filling.

SWEET
PIES

✦ ✦ ✦ ✦ ✦

Strawberry Apple Streusel Pie 37

Raspberry Pie 39

Maple Blueberry Pie 41

Blackberry Streusel Pie 42

Sweetheart Cherry Pie 43

Summer Peach Pie 45

Marionberry Pie with Hazelnut Crust 47

Italian Prune Plum Walnut Cobbler 48

Traditional Apple Pie 50

Blackberry Crumble 51

Winter Pear and Cranberry Streusel Pie 53

✦ ✦ ✦ ✦ ✦

T HE PIES IN THIS CHAPTER ARE THE CLASSIC "home on the range" kind that we Americans have come to know and look forward to with great fondness. They are the pies my mother made so well when I was growing up. On weekends my family spent full days doing chores, gardening, and studying. So it was with great pleasure that we would sit down to a contented dinner followed by a luscious slice of her mouthwatering pie.

With the exception of Italian Prune Plum Walnut Cobbler (page 48), I call for these pies to be made in a 9-inch pan. These are the deeper-dish kind of pies, filled to the brim—and sometimes more so—with seasonal fruits covered by tasty pastry. Please read the tips in the Pastry Doughs chapter (pages 3–6), if you haven't already done so: they're very helpful as you make the crusts for these recipes.

SWEET PIE TIPS AND TECHNIQUES

USING A PREHEATED BAKING PAN OR STONE: For all the pies in this chapter, I recommend that you place an aluminum foil–lined baking sheet or baking stone in the oven as it's preheating. There are two reasons for this. First, the pan will catch any juices that bubble up and drip, making cleanup easier. Second, and more importantly, the hot surface helps ensure a crisp and thoroughly baked bottom crust.

THICKENING THE FILLING: In this book, I call for quick-cooking tapioca, tapioca flour, rice flour, or arrowroot as a thickener for the fruit fillings. I love the way tapioca subtly gels the filling and the way arrowroot and rice flour thicken with a very gentle touch. While some people prefer cornstarch as a thickener because it has no taste, I chose not to use corn in these recipes because many people are allergic to it. If you'd like to use cornstarch instead, the rule of thumb is to substitute the same amount as the thickener I call for. Be sure to let the filling sit for the full amount of time called for in each recipe before pouring into your crust.

BROWNING THE CRUST: As these crusts do not overbrown or burn, it's not necessary to use a pie protector or an aluminum foil tent. However, do bake them on the middle rack of your oven unless specified in the recipe.

SLICING THE PIE: Most of these pies call for a top crust made of wedges that fit together to create a circle. This makes the pies very easy to slice: simply cut between the wedges for a lovely, defined triangular slice. For pies that are decorated with hearts, I make three different sizes of hearts and place the largest ones in a circle on the outside of the pie, followed by the middle-size heart, with the smallest right in the center. This way the hearts are laid out such that you can slice a lovely wedge of pie without slicing into the adorably shaped crusts. Of course, these details are here for those who are concerned with presentation. We all know what matters most with pie is the taste, and on that note, these pies will delight!

✦ Strawberry Apple Streusel Pie ✦

A warm slice of this pie, with its juicy strawberries covering lightly spiced apples under a crisp streusel-like topping, is superbly satisfying. This recipe works beautifully with other berries too, such as a combination of blueberries and blackberries instead of the strawberries.

‖‖‖‖‖‖‖‖‖‖‖‖‖‖‖‖‖‖‖‖‖‖‖‖‖‖‖‖‖ **MAKES ONE 9-INCH PIE** ‖‖‖‖‖‖‖‖‖‖‖‖‖‖‖‖‖‖‖‖‖‖‖‖‖‖‖‖‖‖‖

EQUIPMENT: 9-inch pie pan

1 Single Crust with Streusel Topping (page 16)

1 pound fresh strawberries, hulled and sliced (about 3 cups)

1½ pounds apples, peeled, cored, and sliced

½ cup maple syrup

3 tablespoons quick-cooking tapioca

2 tablespoons tapioca flour

4 teaspoons freshly squeezed lemon juice

1 teaspoon ground cinnamon

1 teaspoon vanilla extract

1. Prepare the crust as instructed.

2. Preheat the oven to 375 degrees F. Place a baking stone or aluminum foil–lined baking sheet on the middle rack of the oven.

3. To make the filling, in a large bowl, combine the remaining ingredients. Let the filling sit for 15 minutes.

4. Spoon the filling into the prepared bottom crust, then evenly sprinkle the streusel over the top.

5. Place the pie on the baking stone or sheet. Bake for 1 hour and 20 minutes, or until the filling is slightly bubbling and the streusel is lightly browned. Let the pie cool for 1 hour before serving.

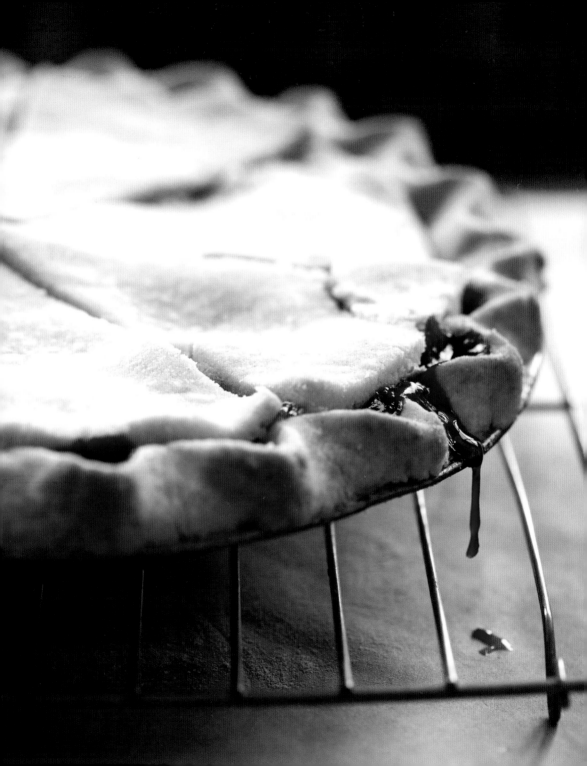

✦ Raspberry Pie ✦

Sitting down to a piece of Raspberry Pie at least once a year is such a treat. After making this pie, you may consider planting some raspberry canes nearby, if you haven't already, as these red jewels cost a pretty penny. For a fun and fancy appearance, use a small, well-floured heart, star, leaf, or circular cookie cutter to remove a small piece out of each wedge in the top crust and expose some of the bright filling.

‖‖‖‖‖‖‖‖‖‖‖‖‖‖‖‖‖‖‖‖‖‖‖‖‖‖‖‖ **MAKES ONE 9-INCH PIE** ‖‖‖‖‖‖‖‖‖‖‖‖‖‖‖‖‖‖‖‖‖‖‖‖‖‖‖‖‖

EQUIPMENT: 9-inch pie pan

1 Double Pastry Crust (page 11) with a wedge top crust

2 tablespoons quick-cooking tapioca

1 tablespoon arrowroot

1 tablespoon freshly squeezed lemon juice

⅔ cup Sucanat or evaporated cane juice

1½ pounds fresh raspberries (about 5 cups)

3 tablespoons seedless raspberry jam

‖‖‖

1. Prepare the crust as instructed.

2. Preheat the oven to 425 degrees F. Place a baking stone or aluminum foil–lined baking sheet on the bottom rack of the oven.

3. In a large bowl, combine the tapioca, arrowroot, lemon juice, and Sucanat. Gently fold in the raspberries, keeping them intact. Let the filling sit for 15 minutes.

4. Spread the raspberry jam over the prepared bottom crust. Pour the filling over the jam, then arrange the top wedge crust.

5. Place the pie on the baking stone or sheet. Bake for 30 minutes, then rotate the pie 180 degrees and reduce the oven temperature to 350 degrees F. Bake for an additional 35 minutes. Let the pie cool for about 1½ hours before serving.

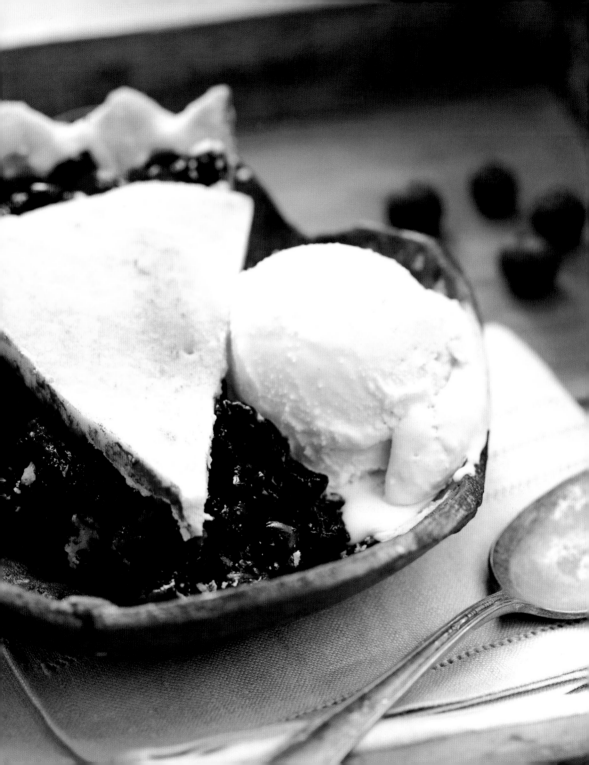

✦ Maple Blueberry Pie ✦

A forkful of fresh blueberries baked with maple syrup, lemon juice, a hint of cinnamon, and a "buttery" crust is a simply mandatory experience. Homemade classic blueberry pie sitting so plump and proudly on the plate delivers sheer exaltation!

||||||||||||||||||||||||||||||||||||||||||| **MAKES ONE 9-INCH PIE** |||||||||||||||||||||||||||||||||||||||||||

EQUIPMENT: 9-inch pie pan

1 Double Pastry Crust (page 11), with a wedge top crust

3 pounds fresh blueberries (about 6 cups)

1 cup maple syrup

⅓ cup quick-cooking tapioca

¼ cup tapioca flour

4 teaspoons freshly squeezed lemon juice

½ teaspoon ground cinnamon

|||||||||||||||||||||||||||||||||||||||||||||||||||||||||||||||||||||||||||||||||||||||||||||||||||||||||||||||||||||||||

1. Prepare the crust as instructed.

2. Preheat the oven to 425 degrees F. Place a baking stone or aluminum foil–lined baking sheet on the middle rack of the oven.

3. To make the filling, in a large bowl, combine the remaining ingredients. Let the filling sit for 15 minutes.

4. Pour the filling into the prepared bottom crust, then arrange the wedge top crust.

5. Place the pie on the baking stone or sheet. Bake for 20 minutes, then rotate the pie 180 degrees and reduce the oven temperature to 375 degrees F. Bake for an additional 1 hour, or until the filling is bubbling and the crust is golden brown. Let the pie cool for about 1½ hours before serving.

✦ Blackberry Streusel Pie ✦

A slice of this blackberry pie, in my opinion, is the most sublime way to conclude a late-summer evening! The crumble topping contrasts in the most enjoyable way with the juicy, slightly sweetened blackberries. I like to prepare a large pitcher of rooibos iced tea to accompany the warm pie. I find the tea's slight apricot flavor pairs harmoniously with the blackberries.

|||||||||||||||||||||||||||||||||||||||||| **MAKES ONE 9-INCH PIE** ||||||||||||||||||||||||||||||||||||||||||

EQUIPMENT: 9-inch pie pan

1 Single Crust with Streusel Topping (page 16)

1½ teaspoons lemon zest

Juice of 1 lemon

½ cup packed dark brown sugar

2 tablespoons quick-cooking tapioca

2 tablespoons arrowroot

2 pounds blackberries (about 6 cups)

|||||||||||||||||||||||||||||||||||||||||||||||||||||||||||||||||||||||||||||||||||||||||||||||||||||||||||||||||||

1. Prepare the crust as instructed.

2. Preheat the oven to 425 degrees F. Place a baking stone or aluminum foil–lined baking sheet on the bottom rack of the oven.

3. In a large bowl, combine the lemon zest and juice, brown sugar, tapioca, and arrowroot. Gently fold in the blackberries, keeping them intact. Let the filling sit for 15 minutes.

4. Spoon the filling into the prepared bottom crust, then evenly sprinkle the streusel over the top.

5. Place the pie on the baking stone or sheet. Bake for 30 minutes, then rotate the pie 180 degrees and reduce the oven temperature to 350 degrees F. Bake for an additional 35 minutes, or until the filling is bubbling and the streusel is golden. Let the pie cool for about 1½ hours before serving.

⋆ Sweetheart Cherry Pie ⋆

I call this pie "Sweetheart," because I love the name of that particular cherry, which is known for its sweetness and firmness. However, I've made this beautiful pie with fresh bing, Lambert, and Rainier cherries, and I can't say that one variety is more delicious than another. You might enjoy experimenting with a combination of cherry types. If you like, use a small, well-floured heart cookie cutter to remove a small piece out of each wedge in the top crust to expose some of the bright filling.

|||||||||||||||||||||||||||||||||||||||||| **MAKES ONE 9-INCH PIE** ||||||||||||||||||||||||||||||||||||||||||||

EQUIPMENT: 9-inch pie pan

1 Double Pastry Crust (page 11) with a wedge top crust

2¼ pounds fresh sweet cherries such as Sweetheart, bing, Lambert, or Rainier, pitted and halved

¼ cup evaporated cane juice

3 tablespoons quick-cooking tapioca

1 tablespoon lemon juice

|||||||||||||||||||||||||||||||||||||||||||||||||||||||||||||||||||||||||||||||||||||||||||||||||||||||||||||||||||

1. Prepare the crust as instructed.

2. Preheat the oven to 400 degrees F. Place a baking stone or aluminum foil–lined baking sheet on the middle rack of the oven.

3. To make the filling, in a large glass or ceramic bowl, combine the remaining ingredients. Let the filling sit for 20 minutes.

4. Pour the filling into the prepared bottom crust, then arrange the wedge top crust.

5. Place the pie on the baking stone or sheet. Bake for 20 minutes, then rotate the pie 180 degrees and reduce the oven temperature to 350 degrees F. Bake for an additional 50 minutes, or until the filling is bubbling and the crust is golden brown. Let the pie cool for about 1½ hours before serving.

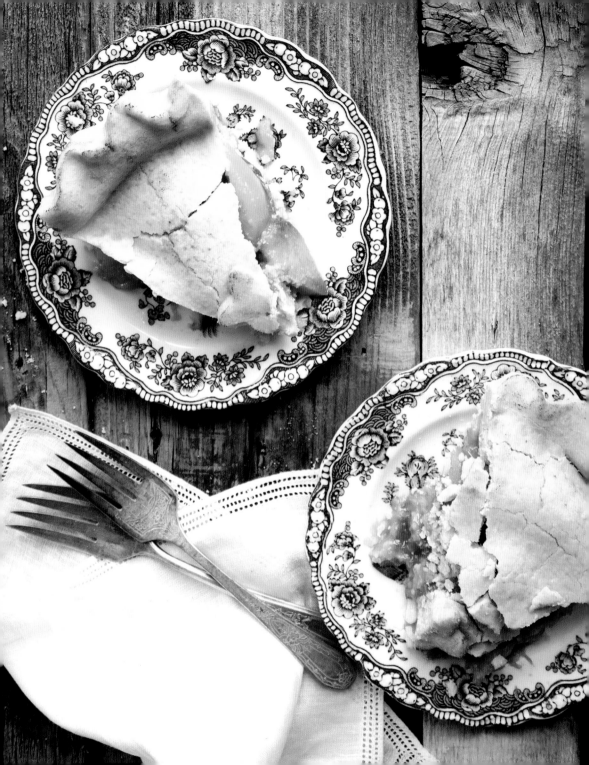

✦ Summer Peach Pie ✦

This peach pie expresses summer at its peak. I adapted this recipe from the inge-nious Rose Levy Beranbaum, who wrote The Pie and Pastry Bible. *I love how the filling is succulent and totally peachy but not overly wet with juice: the secret is cooking down some of the strained peach juices. Feel free to substitute white peaches and/or nectarines, but no matter what you use, make sure they're ripe. Peaches tend to be at their best when they're just slightly soft to the touch.*

In this recipe I call for a traditional top crust that covers the entire pie. If you prefer a wedge top crust, that's a good option as well, as the filling levels smoothly.

||||||||||||||||||||||||||||||||||||| **MAKES ONE 9-INCH PIE** |||||||||||||||||||||||||||||||||||||||||

EQUIPMENT: 9-inch pie pan

1 Double Pastry Crust (page 11) or
  Darker Double Crust (page 14)

2¾ pounds (about 8 medium)
  peaches, blanched, peeled, pitted,
  and sliced ⅛ inch thick

1 tablespoon freshly squeezed
  lemon juice

⅓ cup evaporated cane juice

Pinch of sea salt

2 teaspoons arrowroot

2 teaspoons quick-cooking tapioca

||||||||||||||||||||||||||||||||||||||||||||||||||||||||||||||||||||||||||||||||||||||||||||||||||||||||||||||||

1. Prepare the bottom crust as instructed.

2. In a large bowl, combine the peaches, lemon juice, evaporated cane juice, and sea salt. Let the mixture sit for 30 minutes.

3. Transfer the mixture to a colander placed over a bowl and let the juices drain into the bowl. In a small saucepan over medium heat, cook ⅔ cup of the peach liquid until it becomes syrupy and reduces to about ⅓ cup, about 5 to 7 minutes. Remove the pan from the heat and let the syrup cool.

4. Return the peaches to the large bowl and toss them with the arrowroot and tapioca. Pour the cooled syrup over the peaches and toss again. Let the filling sit for 15 minutes.

continued

5. Spoon the filling into the prepared bottom crust. Roll out the top crust to cover the peach filling: Place the dough on a well-floured, parchment-lined firm piece of cardboard. Roll the dough out to an 11-inch diameter, then gently flip the dough over the filling. Crimp or flute the edges of the dough (see "Fluting the bottom crust," page 5). With a sharp knife, make 5 evenly spaced 2-inch-long slashes in the center of the pie radiating out like the spokes of a wheel. Place the entire pie in the freezer for about 35 minutes.

6. Preheat the oven to 425 degrees F. Place a baking stone or aluminum foil–lined baking sheet on the bottom rack of the oven.

7. Place the pie on the baking stone or sheet. Bake for 50 minutes, or until the filling is bubbling and the crust is golden brown. Let the pie cool for about 2½ hours before serving.

✦ Marionberry Pie with Hazelnut Crust ✦

Crunchy, delicate ground hazelnuts lend their sweetness to the crust, and are simply wonderful with a mouthful of tart-sweet marionberry filling. The top of this hazelnut crust is arranged adorably with pastry cutouts in the shape of hearts!

||||||||||||||||||||||||||||||||||||||||||| **MAKES ONE 9-INCH PIE** |||||||||||||||||||||||||||||||||||||||||||

EQUIPMENT: 9-inch pie pan

1 Hazelnut Pastry Crust (page 18) with heart cutout top crust

⅔ cup evaporated cane juice or Sucanat

2 tablespoons quick-cooking tapioca

1 tablespoon arrowroot

1 tablespoon freshly squeezed lemon juice

Pinch of salt

4½ cups fresh marionberries (about 2 pounds)

||||||||||||||||||||||||||||||||||||||||||||||||||||||||||||||||||||||||||||||||||||||||||||||||||||||||||||||||||||||

1. Prepare the crust as instructed.

2. Preheat the oven to 425 degrees F. Place a baking stone or aluminum foil–lined baking sheet on the bottom rack of the oven.

3. In a large bowl, combine the evaporated cane juice, tapioca, arrowroot, lemon juice, and salt. Gently fold in the marionberries, keeping them intact. Let the filling sit for 15 minutes.

4. Spoon the filling into the prepared bottom crust and then arrange the cutout hearts over the top. Place the larger hearts closer to the edge of the pie and nestle the smaller hearts in the center. You can also alternate the direction of the hearts to fit more crust pieces on top.

5. Place the pie on the baking stone or sheet. Bake for 30 minutes, then rotate the pie 180 degrees and reduce the oven temperature to 375 degrees F. Bake for an additional 35 minutes, or until the filling is bubbling and the crust is golden brown. Let the pie cool for about 1½ hours before serving.

⋅ Italian Prune Plum Walnut Cobbler ⋅

Italian prune plums sprinkled with a smidgen of lemon juice, sweetened with maple syrup, and tucked underneath pastry with toasted walnuts are fabulous. Enjoy this dessert warm, served in bowls, perhaps à la mode. I like to decorate this cobbler with rows of cutout hearts alternating directions, but you can use any shape you like.

||||||||||||||||||||||||||||||||||||| **MAKES ONE 9-BY-13-INCH COBBLER** |||||||||||||||||||||||||||||||||||||

EQUIPMENT: 9-by-13-inch pan

FOR THE DOUGH:

1 cup brown rice flour

¼ cup tapioca flour

½ cup ground toasted walnuts

¼ cup arrowroot

1 tablespoon evaporated cane juice

½ teaspoon baking powder

½ teaspoon ground cinnamon

¼ teaspoon salt

½ cup refined coconut oil

1 tablespoon water

1 teaspoon vanilla extract

FOR THE FILLING:

6 cups halved and pitted fresh Italian prune plums

⅔ cup maple syrup

1 tablespoon freshly squeezed lemon juice

3 tablespoons arrowroot

||||||||||||||||||||||||||||||||||||||||||||||||||||||||||||||||||||||||||||||||||||||||||||||||||||||||||||||||||||

1. Preheat the oven to 375 degrees F.

2. To make the dough, place the flours, walnuts, arrowroot, evaporated cane juice, baking powder, cinnamon, and salt in the bowl of a food processor and process just until the ingredients are combined. Add the coconut oil and pulse until the dough is the consistency of coarse meal with many pearl-size pieces. Add the water and vanilla, and process until the dough holds together.

3. Place the dough on a piece of parchment paper well dusted with brown rice flour. Shape it into a disc with your hands. Dust both your rolling pin and the disc with brown rice flour. Roll the dough out to a ¼-inch thickness. With a cookie cutter or freehand, cut out your favorite shapes, using up all of the dough.

4. To make the filling, in a large bowl, combine the remaining ingredients. Let the filling sit for 15 minutes.

5. Spoon the filling evenly a 9-by-13-inch pan. Top decoratively with the dough pieces. Bake for 1 hour, or until the filling is bubbling and the cobbler crust is golden and firm. Let the pie cool for about 1 hour before serving.

THIS RECIPE HAS BEEN DESIGNED AROUND ITALIAN PRUNE PLUMS, but the combination of nectarines and plums is also remarkably tasty and worth trying. The nectarines add a bright tang and a touch of late summer to the dessert. If using nectarines, slice them into quarters. I am a fan of leaving the skins on. If you prefer peeled fruit, bring a large pot of water to a gentle boil, then prepare an ice bath in a large bowl filled with cold water and ice. Allow your clean plums or nectarines to blanch in the boiling water for approximately 90 seconds. Using a slotted spoon, lift the fruit out of the hot water and transfer to the ice bath to chill for about 5 minutes. With a pairing knife, gently peel back the skins. Set the fruit aside for slicing.

✦ Traditional Apple Pie ✦

I love using a variety of sweet and tart apples when making the filling because it adds complexity to the flavor. Of my favorites, Pink Ladies and Honeycrisp are more tart while Cameo and Ambrosia are on the sweeter side. I'm sure you will enjoy experimenting with some of the varieties unique to your region.

|||||||||||||||||||||||||||||||||||||||||||| **MAKES ONE 9-INCH PIE** ||||||||||||||||||||||||||||||||||||||||||||

EQUIPMENT: 9-inch pie pan

1 Darker Double Crust (page 14)

3 pounds combined sweet and tart
   apples, cored and sliced ¼ inch thick

¾ teaspoon ground cinnamon

2½ tablespoons arrowroot

⅓ cup evaporated cane juice

¼ cup packed dark brown sugar

⅓ cup raisins

1 tablespoon vanilla extract

2 teaspoons lemon juice

¼ teaspoon sea salt

||||||||||||||||||||||||||||||||||||||||||||||||||||||||||||||||||||||||||||||||||||||||||||||||||||||||||||||||||||

1. Prepare the crust as instructed.

2. To make the filling, in a large bowl, combine the remaining ingredients. Let the filling sit for 30 minutes.

3. Spoon the filling into the prepared bottom crust. Roll out the top crust to cover the apple filling: Place dough on a well-floured, parchment-lined firm piece of cardboard. Roll the dough out to a 10-inch diameter, then gently flip the dough over the filling. Crimp or flute the edges of the dough (see "Fluting the bottom crust," page 5). With a sharp knife, make 5 evenly spaced 2-inch-long slashes in the center of the pie radiating out like the spokes of a wheel. Place the entire pie in the freezer for about 35 minutes.

4. Meanwhile, preheat the oven to 425 degrees F. Place a baking stone or aluminum foil–lined baking sheet on the bottom rack of the oven.

5. Place the pie on the baking stone or sheet. Bake for 15 minutes, then rotate the pie 180 degrees and reduce the oven temperature to 350 degrees F. Bake for an additional 1 hour and 10 minutes, or until the filling is bubbling and the crust is golden and firm. Let the pie cool for about 2 hours before serving.

⋆ Blackberry Crumble ⋆

Crisps are yummy, casual, and inviting, plus they're a breeze to whip up, as they require no rolling and fitting of pastry dough. Of course, blackberries are tasty, but I'm extremely fond of them mainly because I can pick them for free (they grow like weeds in the Pacific Northwest, where I live). A combination of blueberries, blackberries, and raspberries is also divine in this recipe.

|||||||||||||||||||||||||||||||||||||||||| **MAKES ONE 9-INCH CRISP** ||||||||||||||||||||||||||||||||||||||||||

EQUIPMENT: 9-inch pie pan

Coconut oil, for greasing the pan

FOR THE FILLING:

2 tablespoons packed dark brown sugar

1 teaspoon lemon zest

1 tablespoon arrowroot

3 pounds fresh blackberries (about 6 cups)

FOR THE TOPPING:

⅔ cup gluten-free oats

½ cup packed dark brown sugar

¼ cup brown rice flour

½ cup olive oil

½ cup finely chopped walnuts

2 teaspoons ground cinnamon

||||||||||||||||||||||||||||||||||||||||||||||||||||||||||||||||||||||||||||||||||||||||||||||||||||||||||||||||

1. Preheat the oven to 350 degrees F. Lightly grease a 9-inch pie pan with coconut oil and set aside.

2. To make the filling, in a medium bowl, combine the brown sugar, lemon zest, and arrowroot. Gently fold in the blackberries, keeping them intact.

3. To make the topping, in another medium bowl, thoroughly combine the remaining ingredients.

4. Pour the filling into the prepared pie pan, then evenly sprinkle the topping over the filling.

5. Bake for 40 minutes, or until the topping is golden brown and the filling is bubbling. Let the pie cool for about 1 hour before serving.

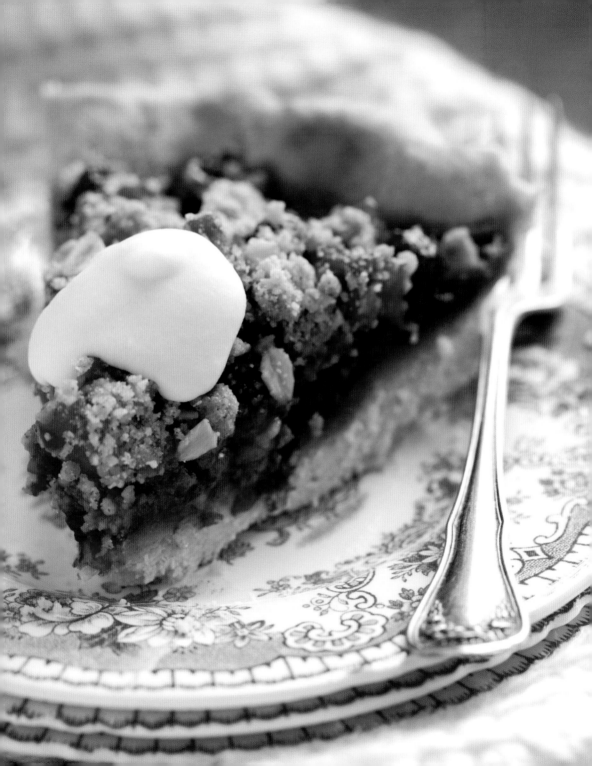

◆ Winter Pear and Cranberry Streusel Pie ◆

I miss fresh berries in the winter, and frozen berries just don't cut it. For me, the combination of sweet pears and plump, tart cranberries, baked with a bit of brown sugar, brings about a dazzling winter metamorphosis. With a slice of this pie before me, I no longer pine for peaches, nectarines, and berries.

|||||||||||||||||||||||||||||||||||||||||||||| **MAKES ONE 9-INCH PIE** ||||||||||||||||||||||||||||||||||||||||||||||

EQUIPMENT: 9-inch pie pan

1 Single Crust with Streusel Topping
  (page 16)

2 large D'Anjou pears, peeled, cored, and cut into ½-inch slices (about 3 cups)

2 cups fresh cranberries

⅔ cup packed dark brown sugar

2½ tablespoons arrowroot

½ teaspoon ground cinnamon

¼ teaspoon ground ginger

⅛ teaspoon ground nutmeg

||||||||||||||||||||||||||||||||||||||||||||||||||||||||||||||||||||||||||||||||||||||||||||||||||||||||||||||||||||||||||||||

1. Prepare the crust as instructed.

2. Preheat the oven to 350 degrees F. Place a baking stone or aluminum foil–lined baking sheet on the middle rack of the oven.

3. To make the filling, in a large bowl, combine the remaining ingredients.

4. Spoon the filling into the prepared bottom crust, then evenly sprinkle the streusel over the top.

5. Place the pie on the baking stone or sheet. Bake for 1 hour, or until the filling is bubbling and the streusel is lightly browned. Let the pie cool for about 1 hour before serving.

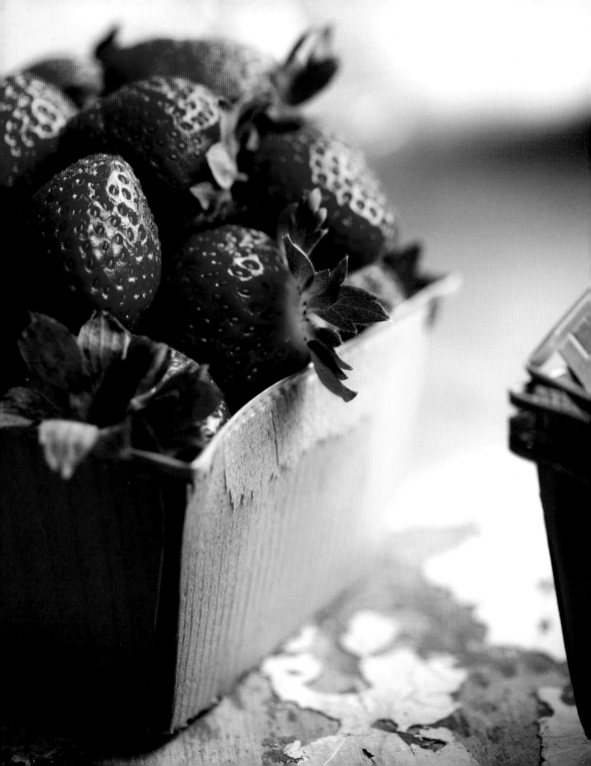

FREE-FORM
PIES

◆ ◆ ◆ ◆ ◆

◆ ◆ ◆ ◆ ◆

FREE-FORM PIES ARE WONDERFULLY TASTY, and their sculptural shapes of folded pastry supporting artfully arranged slices of brightly colored fruits certainly entice. Galettes, crostatas, and croustades conjure up fields of lavender, burnt grass, sturdy old wooden tables, rustic grace, and leisurely long lunches. When I bake one of these special pies, I feel as though I'm entering into a story, bringing a bit of another time into my life.

These pies are easy to create. Arranging sliced fruit in concentric circles is a breeze, and folding the pastry up over the edges of the fruit is simpler than wrapping a gift, yet the finished product gives the impression of artistry. It feels spectacular to see simple pastry and fruit transform into a mouthwatering thing of beauty.

FREE-FORM PIE TIPS AND TECHNIQUES

CUTTING THE FRUIT: Try to slice the fruit uniformly. When the pieces are similar and close in size, the visual effect of the arranged fruit is more striking.

ARRANGING THE FRUIT: For circular pies, locate the central point and, using a ruler or tape measure, measure outward to ensure you leave the border called for in the recipe. Once you have an outline of where the fruit will go, then you can begin overlapping the fruit in either straight rows in the case of the rectangular galette, or in concentric circles for the other pies, starting at the outside of the circle and working toward the center.

FOLDING THE DOUGH: When folding the dough up over the fruit, make sure your hands are clean, dry, and lightly dusted with brown rice flour. If the dough tears, gently mend it by pressing the dough back together with your hands.

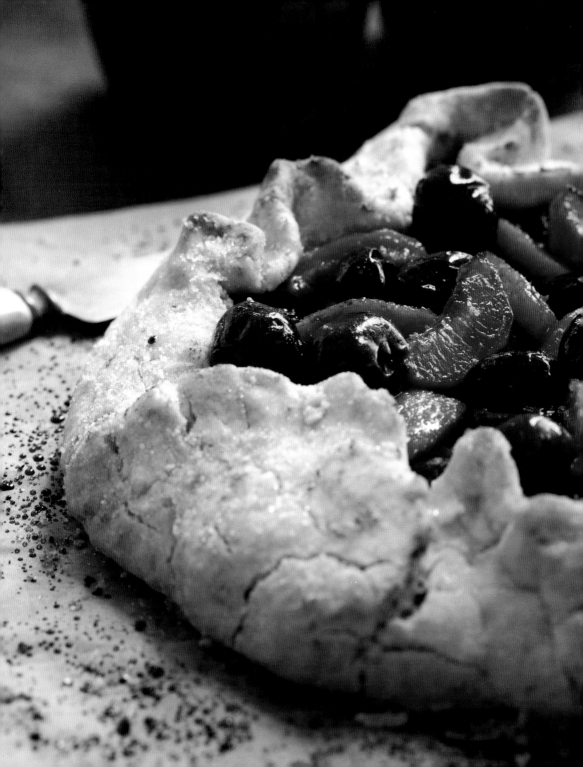

✦ Apricot and Cherry Crostata ✦

In season simultaneously and both so exquisite in taste and color, apricots and cherries baked together create a melody of flavor that is sweet, tart, and tangy. I brush this crostata with warm apricot preserves after it bakes, giving it a finish that's a still life artist's dream. You can make this up to four hours ahead of serving and let it stand at room temperature.

||||||||||||||||||||||||||||||||||| MAKES ONE 13-INCH ROUND CROSTATA |||||||||||||||||||||||||||||||||||

EQUIPMENT: Rimless baking sheet, removable bottom from a tart pan

1 Single Pastry Crust dough (page 9), prepared through Step 1 only

FOR THE FILLING:
8 apricots

2 tablespoons brown rice flour

4 tablespoons evaporated cane juice, divided

1 cup cherries, pitted and halved

2 teaspoons turbinado sugar

¼ cup amount apricot preserves, for brushing (optional)

||||||||||||||||||||||||||||||||||||||||||||||||||||||||||||||||||||||||||||||||||||||||||||||||||||||||||||||||||||||

1. Prepare the dough as instructed.

2. Preheat the oven to 400 degrees F.

3. Set a medium bowl of ice water in the sink. Cook the apricots in a pot of boiling water for 1 to 2 minutes. Using a slotted spoon, transfer the apricots to the ice water. When the apricots have cooled, about 5 minutes, peel, halve, and pit them. Cut each apricot half into 3 wedges.

4. Place the dough on a piece of parchment paper well dusted with brown rice flour. Shape it into a disc with your hands. Dust both your rolling pin and the disc with brown rice flour. As you roll out the dough, rotate the paper so you roll in different directions to produce a 13-inch circle. Transfer the dough, on the parchment paper, to a rimless baking sheet.

5. Combine the brown rice flour with 1 tablespoon of the evaporated cane juice and sprinkle this mixture over the dough. Arrange the apricot wedges, rounded side

continued

down, in overlapping concentric circles, leaving a 3-inch border around the edge of the dough. Place the cherries over and around the apricots. Sprinkle the remaining 3 tablespoons evaporated cane juice over the fruit.

6. Working in 2-inch-wide intervals, fold the border of the dough 2 inches up over the fruit. Leave the center 6 inches of fruit uncovered. Sprinkle the turbinado sugar over the fruit.

7. Bake the crostata until the apricots are tender, about 50 minutes. Use a large spatula to loosen it from the parchment paper, then slide the bottom of a tart pan underneath the crostata to transfer it to a serving platter.

8. Melt the preserves in a small heavy saucepan over low heat, stirring occasionally. Strain into a small bowl through a fine mesh sieve. Brush the strained preserves over the fruit with a small pastry brush; the finish will be glossy and slightly gelled. Serve the crostata slightly warm or at room temperature.

✦ Nectarine and Blackberry Galette ✦

My family has a lot of picnic dinners in the summertime, and this is one of the pies I often pack. I usually slide it onto a tart pan bottom and cover it securely with aluminum foil for the ride. Sweet orange nectarines united with tangy, dark purple blackberries is a marriage made in heaven.

|||||||||||||||||||||||||||||||||||||| **MAKES ONE 12-INCH ROUND GALETTE** ||||||||||||||||||||||||||||||||||||||

EQUIPMENT: Rimless baking sheet removable bottom from a tart pan

1 Single Pastry Crust dough (page 9), prepared through Step 1 only

¼ cup evaporated cane juice or Sucanat

1½ teaspoons arrowroot

3 medium nectarines, pitted and cut into 6 slices each

½ pound blackberries (about 1 cup)

1 tablespoon turbinado sugar

¼ cup peach or apricot preserves (optional)

|||||||||||||||||||||||||||||||||||||||||||||||||||||||||||||||||||||||||||||||||||||||||||||||||||||||||||||||||||||||||||||

1. Prepare the dough as instructed.

2. Preheat the oven to 375 degrees F.

3. Combine the evaporated cane juice and arrowroot in the medium bowl. Gently fold in the nectarines and blackberries. Let the fruit stand, stirring occasionally, until the juices are released, about 30 minutes.

4. Meanwhile, place the dough on a piece of parchment paper well dusted with brown rice flour. Shape it into a disc with your hands. Dust both your rolling pin and the disc with brown rice flour. As you roll out the dough, rotate the paper so you roll in different directions to produce a 12-inch circle. Transfer the dough, on the parchment paper, to a rimless baking sheet.

5. Arrange the fruit in overlapping concentric circles, leaving a 3-inch border around the edge of the dough, and drizzle the juices over the fruit.

continued

6. Working in 2-inch-long intervals, fold the border of the dough 2 inches up over the fruit. Leave the center 6 inches of fruit uncovered. Sprinkle the turbinado sugar over the fruit.

7. Bake the galette for 55 minutes, or until the crust is golden brown and the filling is bubbling. Use a large spatula to loosen it from the parchment paper, then slide the bottom of a tart pan underneath the galette to transfer it to a serving platter.

8. Melt the preserves in a small heavy saucepan over low heat, stirring occasionally. Strain through a fine mesh sieve into a small bowl. Brush the strained preserves over the fruit with a small pastry brush; the finish will be glossy and slightly gelled. Serve the galette warm or at room temperature.

✦ Plum Galette ✦

This galette was inspired by a Martha Stewart recipe. The toasted hazelnuts and baked plum wedges are just right together inside the crisp pastry. I like it to be a bit more tart than my husband would prefer; we've made it with varying amounts of sweetness, and it's always been lovely.

IIIIIIIIIIIIIIIIIIIIIIIIIIIIIIIIIIIII **MAKES ONE 12-BY-16-INCH GALETTE** IIIIIIIIIIIIIIIIIIIIIIIIIIIIIIIII

EQUIPMENT: rimless baking sheet, removable bottom from a tart pan

1 Double Pastry Crust dough (page 11) or Darker Double Crust dough (page 14), prepared through Step 1 only

1 tablespoon brown rice flour

¾ cup finely ground toasted hazelnuts, divided

1½ tablespoons packed dark brown sugar

1 tablespoon arrowroot

¼ teaspoon salt

1½ pounds plums (about 6), pitted and sliced ½ inch thick

2 to 4 tablespoons evaporated cane juice, depending on the level of sweetness you like

⅓ cup red currant or apricot jam (optional)

IIIIIIIIIIIIIIIIIIIIIIIIIIIIIIIIIIIIIIIIIIIIIIIIIIIIIIIIIIIIIIIIIIIIIIIIIIIIIIIIIIIIIIIIIIIIIIIIIIIIIIIIIIIIIIIIIIIIIIIIIIIIII

1. Prepare the dough as instructed.

2. Place the dough on a rimless baking sheet well dusted with brown rice flour. Shape it into a disc with your hands. Dust both your rolling pin and the disc with brown rice flour. Roll the dough out into a 12-by-16-inch rectangle directly on the sheet.

3. In a medium bowl, combine the brown rice flour, ½ cup of the hazelnuts, brown sugar, arrowroot, and salt. Spread this mixture evenly over the dough, leaving a 3-inch border around the edge.

4. Arrange the plums, slightly overlapping, in 4 rows on top of the hazelnut mixture, alternating the direction of the fruit from one row to the next. Sprinkle the evaporated cane juice over the plums. Fold the border of the dough up over the fruit,

continued

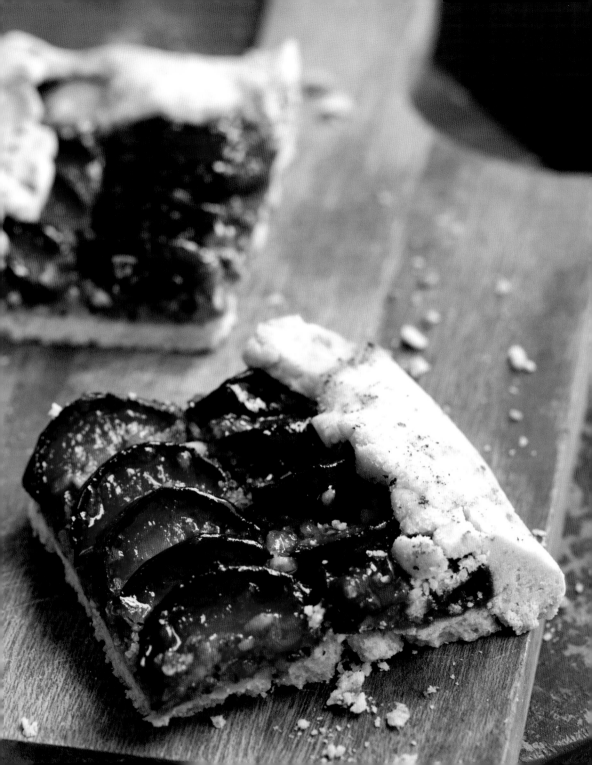

leaving the center uncovered. I like to press a large knife against all 4 sides for a neat look, but you can leave the galette as is. Sprinkle the remaining ¼ cup hazelnuts over the fruit. Place the galette, uncovered, in the refrigerator for about 30 minutes.

5. Meanwhile, preheat the oven to 425 degrees F.

6. Bake the galette for 10 minutes, then reduce the oven temperature to 400 degrees F. Bake for an additional 35 minutes, or until the exposed crust is golden brown and the filling is bubbling.

7. Let the galette cool for 30 minutes. Use a large spatula to loosen it from the baking sheet, then slide the bottom of a tart pan underneath the galette to transfer it to a serving platter.

8. Melt the jam in a small heavy saucepan over low heat, stirring occasionally. Strain through a fine mesh sieve into a small bowl. Brush the strained preserves over the fruit with a small pastry brush; the finish will be glossy and slightly gelled. Serve the galette warm or at room temperature.

✦ Maple-Roasted Peach and Almond Croustade ✦

This free-form croustade is so much fun to create, and its rustic elegance makes quite a welcoming impression. The slivered almonds impart a delicate crunch, in pleasurable contrast to the soft maple-roasted peaches. Enjoy warm, perhaps with a scoop of ice cream.

|||||||||||||||||||||||||||||||| **MAKES ONE 12-INCH ROUND CROUSTADE** ||||||||||||||||||||||||||||||||

EQUIPMENT: rimless baking sheet, removable bottom from a tart pan

1 Single Pastry Crust dough (page 9), prepared through Step 1 only

1½ pounds (about 7) small yellow peaches peeled, quartered, and pitted

4 tablespoons maple syrup, divided

2 tablespoons packed dark brown sugar

¾ cup slivered almonds, divided

2 tablespoons maple syrup

|||||||||||||||||||||||||||||||||||||||||||||||||||||||||||||||||||||||||||||||||||||||||||||||||||||||||||||

1. Prepare the dough as instructed.

2. Preheat the oven to 400 degrees F. Line a baking sheet with aluminum foil. Place the peaches on the foil and drizzle with 2 tablespoons of the maple syrup. Sprinkle the peaches with the brown sugar. Roast the peaches for 20 minutes, then flip them so they brown evenly, and roast for an additional 15 minutes. Set the peaches aside to cool. Reduce the oven temperature to 375 degrees F.

3. Place the dough on a piece of parchment paper well dusted with brown rice flour. Shape it into a disc with your hands. Dust both your rolling pin and the disc with brown rice flour. As you roll out the dough, rotate the paper so you roll in different directions to produce a 12-inch circle. Transfer the dough, on the parchment paper, to a rimless baking sheet.

4. Sprinkle the dough with ½ cup of the almonds. Arrange the peaches in overlapping concentric circles, leaving a 2-inch border around the edge.

5. Working in 2-inch-long intervals, fold the crust 2 inches up over the peaches, then drizzle with the remaining 2 tablespoons maple syrup. Sprinkle the remaining ¼ cup almonds over the crust and fruit. Bake the croustade for 40 minutes, or until the exposed crust is golden brown and the filling is bubbling.

6. Let the croustade cool for 30 minutes. Use a large spatula to loosen it from the parchment paper, then slide the bottom of a tart pan underneath the croustade to transfer it to a serving platter. Serve warm.

✦ Spiced Pear and Hazelnut Croustade ✦

This is an excellent winter treat, with warming, aromatic spices to enliven your spirit on a cold and cloudy day. When I serve this for an afternoon pick-me-up, I also pour piping hot cups of coffee with cardamom; grind the cardamom with your coffee beans before brewing.

||||||||||||||||||||||||||||||| **MAKES ONE 13-INCH ROUND CROUSTADE** |||||||||||||||||||||||||||||||

EQUIPMENT: rimless baking sheet, removable bottom from a tart pan

1 Single Pastry Crust dough (page 9), prepared through Step 1 only

FOR THE FILLING:
2 pounds D'Anjou pears (about 4 medium), peeled, cored, and each cut into 8 wedges

4 tablespoons evaporated cane juice

1 tablespoon brown rice flour

¾ teaspoon ground cardamom

½ teaspoon ground cinnamon

⅛ teaspoon ground cloves

¾ cup coarsely chopped hazelnuts, divided

1 tablespoon evaporated cane juice

||||||||||||||||||||||||||||||||||||||||||||||||||||||||||||||||||||||||||||||||||||||||||||||||||||||||||||||||||||||||||||

1. Prepare the dough as instructed.

2. Preheat the oven to 375 degrees F.

3. In a large bowl, combine the pears with 3 tablespoons of the evaporated cane juice, brown rice flour, cardamom, cinnamon, and cloves; set aside.

4. Place the dough on a piece of parchment paper well dusted with brown rice flour. Shape it into a disc with your hands. Dust both your rolling pin and the disc with brown rice flour. As you roll out the dough, rotate the paper so you roll in different directions to produce a 13-inch circle. Transfer the dough, on the parchment paper, to a rimless baking sheet.

5. Sprinkle the dough with ½ cup of the hazelnuts. Arrange the pears in overlapping concentric circles, leaving a 2-inch border around the edge. Working in 2-inch-long intervals, fold the border of the dough 2 inches up over the pears. Sprinkle the remaining ¼ cup hazelnuts and 1 tablespoon evaporated cane juice.

Bake the croustade for 1 hour, or until the exposed crust is golden brown and the filling is bubbling.

6. Let the croustade cool for 30 minutes. Use a large spatula to loosen it from the parchment paper, then slide the bottom of a tart pan underneath the croustade to transfer it to a serving platter. Serve warm.

HERE'S A LITTLE TRICK FOR PEELING PEARS: USE A POTATO PEELER! You can preserve the shape of the pear and retain more of the fruit while using a peeler rather than a paring knife.

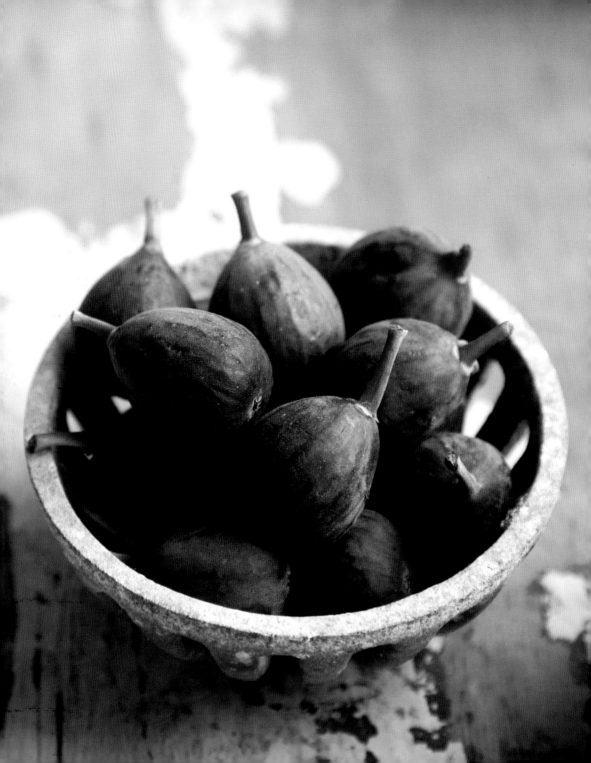

TARTS

◆ ◆ ◆ ◆ ◆

◆ ◆ ◆ ◆ ◆

T

ARTS HOLD A DISTINGUISHED AND CELEBRATED place at the table, so it may surprise you to learn that these exquisite open-faced pies are a cinch to make. In fact, out of all the different pies in this book, tarts are the easiest, after pies with a streusel topping. Here are a few tips to aid you in the tart-making process.

TART TIPS AND TECHNIQUES

TRANSFERRING THE DOUGH TO THE TART PAN: Most of the crusts called for in these recipes are crusts that you simply press into the pan. However, in some recipes, I give you the option of using a Single Pastry Crust (page 9), which, being a rolled-out crust, can be tricky to transfer to a tart pan. You have two options: 1. After you roll out the dough on parchment paper, you can slide the removable bottom of your tart pan under the dough, lifting the dough off the parchment paper in the process. Then drop the pan bottom into the pan's fluted rim and press into place. 2. You can also flip the dough into the pan as described in "Flipping the rolled-out bottom crust into the pan," page 4.

REPAIRING TEARS IN THE DOUGH: If you tear it, the dough is easily mended by pressing it back together with your fingers in your tart pan.

PREPARING FRUIT FILLINGS: Because tarts have no top crust, the more uniformly you can slice the fruit, the more mesmerizing the finished tart will appear.

STORING THE TART: If you won't be enjoying the tart right away, cover it loosely with parchment or waxed paper and refrigerate until serving. Reglaze if needed before slicing. The tarts can be stored up to three days.

✦ Strawberry Rhubarb Tart ✦

Rose Levy Beranbaum, author of The Pie and Pastry Bible, *inspired this gorgeous tart, in which cooked rhubarb filling sits underneath a layer of sliced ripe strawberries. The tart is exquisite to behold and bursts with bright flavor.*

||||||||||||||||||||||||||||||||||||||||| **MAKES ONE 9-INCH TART** |||||||||||||||||||||||||||||||||||||||||

EQUIPMENT: 9-inch fluted round tart pan with a removable bottom

1 Almond Press-In Crust (page 26), Olive Oil Press-In Crust (page 31), Dark Chocolate Pecan Press-In Crust (page 30), Chocolate Almond Press-In Crust (page 27), or Ginger Pecan Press-In Crust (page 28). Or use a Single Pastry Crust (page 9), baked for 40 minutes at 350 degrees F

FOR THE FILLING:

1¼ pounds rhubarb, cut into ½-inch pieces (about 3½ cups)

½ cup evaporated cane juice

Pinch of salt

1 tablespoon arrowroot

⅓ cup currant jelly

12 ounces fresh strawberries, sliced (about 2 cups)

||||||||||||||||||||||||||||||||||||||||||||||||||||||||||||||||||||||||||||||||||||||||||||||||||||||||||||||||||

1. Prepare the crust as instructed.

2. In a large bowl, combine the rhubarb, evaporated cane juice, salt, and arrowroot, and let sit for 15 minutes, or until the rhubarb becomes juicy.

3. In a large saucepan over medium heat, bring the rhubarb mixture to a boil, stirring continuously. Reduce the heat to a low simmer and cover the pan. Cook the rhubarb until it has softened, about 10 minutes, stirring it every few minutes. Remove the pan from the heat and let the rhubarb cool for about 1 hour.

4. In a small saucepan, warm the jelly over low heat until it's just slightly melted. Strain through a fine mesh sieve into a small bowl. Brush the tart crust with some of the strained jelly, reserving the majority for the strawberries. Pour the rhubarb mixture into the crust, smoothing the top. Arrange the strawberries in concentric circles over the rhubarb, then brush them with the remaining strained jelly, rewarming it if needed to make it spreadable.

✦ Fresh Fruit Tart ✦

Topped with glistening fresh kiwis, raspberries, and blueberries, this tart really shines for brunch, a fancy luncheon, or a romantic dessert. A smidgen of brandy in the cream filling makes for a delightful zing. Feel free to substitute other fruit, such as strawberries, mangoes, peaches, or blackberries.

|||||||||||||||||||||||||||||||||||||| **MAKES ONE 10-INCH TART** ||||||||||||||||||||||||||||||||||||||||

EQUIPMENT: 10-inch fluted round tart pan with a removable bottom

1 Almond Press-In Crust (page 26), Dark Chocolate Pecan Press-In Crust (page 30), Chocolate Almond Press-In Crust (page 27), or Ginger Pecan Press-In Crust (page 28). Or use a Single Pastry Crust (page 9), baked for 40 minutes at 350 degrees F

FOR THE FILLING:

¼ cup raw cashews, soaked in water for 2 to 8 hours (see "Soaking the cashews," page 106) and drained

¾ cup coconut milk

1½ teaspoons vanilla extract

1 tablespoon brandy

2 tablespoons water

2 teaspoons agar flakes

2 tablespoons maple syrup

1½ tablespoons coconut oil

FOR THE TOPPING:

2 large kiwis, peeled, halved lengthwise, and sliced

6 ounces fresh raspberries (about 1 cup)

8 ounces fresh blueberries (about 1 cup)

¼ cup apple jelly or apricot jam, for glazing

|||||||||||||||||||||||||||||||||||||||||||||||||||||||||||||||||||||||||||||||||||||||||||||||||||||||||

1. Prepare the crust as instructed.

2. Place the in a blender or the bowl of a food processor along with the coconut milk, vanilla, and brandy. Process thoroughly until very creamy and smooth. Leave the mixture in the blender.

3. To make the filling, in a small saucepan, stir together the water, agar, and maple syrup. Bring the mixture to a boil, then reduce the heat to a simmer. Simmer for 3 minutes, stirring occasionally, then remove the pan from the heat and stir in the

continued

coconut oil. Add the mixture to the cashew mixture in the blender and process until thoroughly incorporated and smooth.

4. Pour the filling evenly into the crust and refrigerate for 2 hours. After the filling has set, decoratively arrange the kiwis, raspberries, and blueberries on top. I like to place the kiwis around the outside of the tart, followed by a circle of the blueberries and finishing with the raspberries in the center.

5. In a small saucepan, warm the jelly over low heat until it's just slightly melted. Strain through a fine mesh sieve into a small bowl. Brush the strained jelly over the fruit with a small pastry brush; the finish will be glossy and slightly gelled. Serve immediately.

• Autumn Tart •

A mélange of autumn fruits are deliciously baked together in this lightly maple-sweetened tart with a surprising yet mellow hint of rich balsamic vinegar. I especially enjoy this tart with the Canola Oil Walnut Press-In Crust (page 32).

||||||||||||||||||||||||||||||||||||||||||| **MAKES ONE 9-INCH TART** |||||||||||||||||||||||||||||||||||||||||||

EQUIPMENT: 9-inch fluted round tart pan with a removable bottom

1 Canola Oil Walnut Press-In Crust (page 32).

FOR THE FILLING:

2 red plums, pitted and cut into 6 wedges each

1 red apple, cored and cut into ¼-inch slices

1 pear, cored and cut into ¼-inch slices

1 pound fresh blackberries, raspberries, or elderberries

½ teaspoon ground cinnamon

3 tablespoons maple syrup

1 tablespoon balsamic vinegar

3 tablespoons apricot jam (optional)

|||||||||||||||||||||||||||||||||||||||||||||||||||||||||||||||||||||||||||||||||||||||||||||||||||||||||||||||||||||||||||||

1. Prepare the crust as instructed.

2. Preheat the oven to 350 degrees F.

3. In a large bowl, combine the plums, apple, pear, berries, cinnamon, maple syrup, and balsamic vinegar. Toss the fruit gently to coat.

4. Arrange the fruit slices decoratively in concentric circles on the crust, scattering the berries over the top of the other fruit.

5. Bake the tart for 1 hour and 20 minutes. Let the tart cool 1 hour

6. Once the tart has cooled, warm the jam in a small saucepan until it is slightly melted. Strain through a fine mesh sieve into a small bowl. Brush the strained jam over the fruit with a small pastry brush; the finish will be glossy and slightly gelled. Serve warm.

✦ Fig Frangipane Tart ✦

I am particularly dazzled by the beauty of a sliced fresh fig. This tart shows them off stunningly, quartered and arranged in a circular pattern. Being so exceptionally sweet on their own, figs require very little additional sugar. Set in an almond custard-like cream atop a crisp and tender crust, they are extra delicious.

|||||||||||||||||||||||||||||||||||||||||||||||||| **MAKES ONE 10-INCH TART** ||||||||||||||||||||||||||||||||||||||||||||||||||

EQUIPMENT: 10-inch fluted round tart pan with a removable bottom

1 Single Pastry Crust (page 9), baked
for 40 minutes at 350 degrees F

FOR THE FILLING:

1 cup whole blanched almonds,
toasted and cooled

⅓ cup plus 2 tablespoons evaporated
cane juice, divided

5 tablespoons olive oil

½ cup almond milk

2 tablespoons arrowroot

1½ teaspoons vanilla extract

Pinch of sea salt

8 fresh figs, stemmed and quartered

1 tablespoon turbinado sugar

|||||||||||||||||||||||||||||||||||||||||||||||||||||||||||||||||||||||||||||||||||||||||||||||||||||||||||||||||||||||||||||||||||

1. Prepare the crust as instructed.

2. Preheat the oven to 375 degrees F.

3. In the bowl of a food processor, combine the almonds and 2 tablespoons of the evaporated cane juice. Pulse until the almonds are finely ground, then add the remaining ⅓ cup evaporated cane juice, olive oil, almond milk, arrowroot, vanilla, and sea salt. Process thoroughly until very creamy and smooth.

4. Pour the filling into the prebaked crust and smooth the top. Arrange the figs in a decorative circular pattern over the filling. Sprinkle with the turbinado sugar and bake for 45 minutes. Let the tart cool for 1 hour before serving.

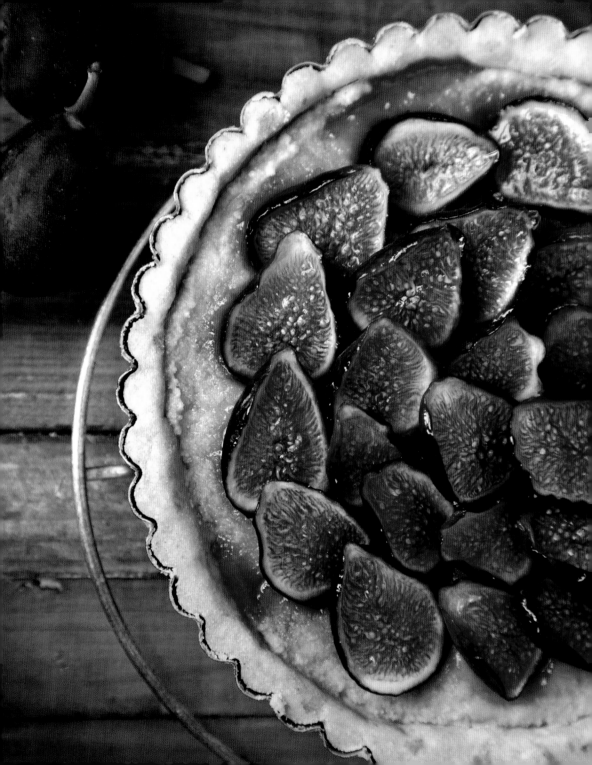

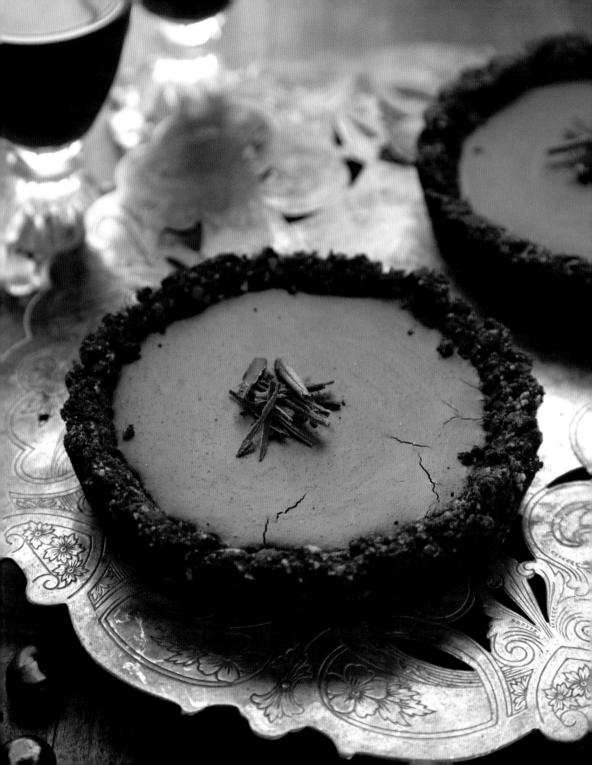

✦ Chocolate Espresso Tart ✦

It's no secret that dark chocolate and coffee make a formidable marriage as far as taste buds are concerned. This particular tart is so smooth, the filling reminds me of a truffle. A word of caution: If you're sensitive to caffeine, I advise enjoying this decadent dessert after lunch as opposed to after dinner. Otherwise you may find yourself wide awake into the wee hours of the morning. Enjoy a rich sliver accompanied by a hot drink or a glass of red wine.

||||||||||||||||||||||||||||||||||||||||| **MAKES ONE 9-INCH TART** |||||||||||||||||||||||||||||||||||||||||||||||

EQUIPMENT: 9-inch fluted round tart pan with a removable bottom

1 Canola Oil Walnut Press-In Crust (page 32), Olive Oil Press-In Crust (page 31), Dark Chocolate Pecan Press-In Crust (page 30), or Chocolate Almond Press-In Crust (page 27). Or use a Single Pastry Crust (page 9), baked for 40 minutes at 350 degrees F

FOR THE FILLING:

5.3 ounces 72% dark baking chocolate, broken into pieces

⅔ cup coconut oil

1 teaspoon vanilla extract

⅛ teaspoon salt

¼ cup brewed espresso (espresso is ideal, but coffee will work)

Chocolate shavings, for garnish

Chocolate-covered espresso beans, for garnish

||||||||||||||||||||||||||||||||||||||||||||||||||||||||||||||||||||||||||||||||||||||||||||||||||||||||||||||||||||||||||||||||||

1. Prepare the crust as instructed.

2. Melt the chocolate over low heat in a double boiler or a stainless steel bowl set over a small saucepan filled with about 2 inches of gently simmering water. (The bowl should not touch the water.) Remove the pan from the heat and mix in the coconut oil, vanilla, salt, and espresso. Let the mixture sit for 30 minutes; it will thicken. Pour the filling into the crust and smooth the type. Refrigerate the tart for 30 minutes. When the filling has set, garnish with the chocolate shavings and/or the espresso beans.

✦ Chocolate Prune Tart ✦

I created this tart for my dear friend Gabrielle on her birthday. It's rich, delicious, and robust with antioxidants, with only a modest amount of sweetener. I particularly enjoy it with the Dark Chocolate Pecan Press-In Crust (page 30).

|||||||||||||||||||||||||||||||||||||||||||||| **MAKES ONE 9-INCH TART** ||||||||||||||||||||||||||||||||||||||||||||||

EQUIPMENT: 9-inch fluted round tart pan with a removable bottom

1 Canola Oil Walnut Press-In Crust (page 32), Olive Oil Press-In Crust (page 31), Dark Chocolate Pecan Press-In Crust (page 30), or Chocolate Almond Press-In Crust (page 27). Or use a Single Pastry Crust (page 9), baked for 40 minutes at 350 degrees F

⅔ cup pitted prunes

4 ounces unsweetened baking chocolate

3 tablespoons coconut oil

1 teaspoon vanilla extract

¼ cup maple syrup

2 tablespoons Grand Marnier

⅛ teaspoon salt

Dark chocolate shavings or curls, for garnish (optional)

Sliced strawberries, for garnish (optional)

||||||||||||||||||||||||||||||||||||||||||||||||||||||||||||||||||||||||||||||||||||||||||||||||||||||||||||||||||||||||||||||||||

1. Prepare the crust as instructed.

2. Place the prunes in a small saucepan and cover with water. Bring the water to a boil, then reduce the heat to a simmer. Cover the pan and let the prunes simmer for 30 minutes, or until soft. Drain the prunes, reserving 1 tablespoon of the prune water; set aside.

3. Melt the chocolate over low heat in a double boiler or a stainless steel bowl set over a small saucepan filled with about 2 inches of gently simmering water. (The bowl should not touch the water.)

4. In the bowl of a food processor, process the melted chocolate, prunes and reserved water, coconut oil, vanilla, maple syrup, Grand Marnier, and salt until the mixture has a smooth, pudding-like consistency.

5. Pour the filling into the crust and smooth the top. Refrigerate the tart for 2 hours. After the filling has set, garnish with dark chocolate shavings and/or strawberries. Serve at room temperature.

⁕ Linzer Torte ⁕

This torte is visually impressive with its lattice top. The ground hazelnuts add their own particular sweetness. The pastry, having a touch of rising agent, is a tad more cookielike than the other crusts in this book. If you're intimidated by gluten-free lattice crusts, then this is a marvelous recipe to dive into, as the diamond pattern I use doesn't require you to weave the dough. You can experiment with a variety of jam fillings.

|||||||||||||||||||||||||||||||||||||||||||| **MAKES ONE 10-INCH TORTE** ||||||||||||||||||||||||||||||||||||||||||||

EQUIPMENT: 10-inch round tart pan or springform pan, rimless baking sheet

1 Hazelnut Pastry Crust dough (page 18), prepared through Step 2 only

1 cup bilberry jam

1. Prepare the crust as instructed.

2. Preheat the oven to 350 degrees F.

3. Place the dough on a piece of parchment paper well dusted with brown rice flour. Divide it into two portions, one slightly larger (about two-thirds of the dough) than the other; this will be the bottom crust. Roll the smaller portion out into a 10-inch circle (the bottom of your springform or tart pan will be an excellent template). Using a sharp knife, slice the circle into ten ½-inch strips.

4. Use the parchment paper to transfer the strips to a rimless baking sheet or cutting board (whichever fits more easily into your freezer) by sliding the sheet under the parchment paper. Gently separate each strip of dough with a knife so that the pieces do not stick together during freezing. Place the baking sheet, uncovered, in the freezer for 15 minutes, or until the dough is firm. Using the scrap dough, create leaves to cover the perimeter of the torte after the strips have been arranged.

5. Press the larger portion of dough into the tart pan. The dough should rise about ¼ inch up the side of the pan. Spread the jam evenly over the crust. Place 5 dough

continued

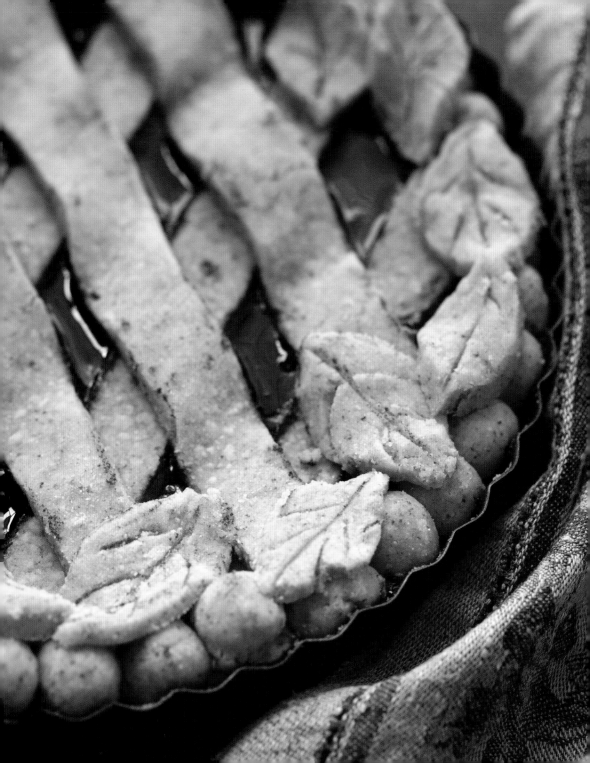

strips across the pan, spacing them evenly. Give the pan a quarter turn and lay the remaining strips across the first 5. Trim any excess dough from the strips and use them to make more leaves if needed. Place the dough leaves around the outside of the torte. Bake for 35 minutes, or until the tart is golden and the filling is bubbling.

BILBERRY FRUIT IS VERY SIMILAR TO OUR BELOVED BLUEBERRY! It may be of interest to know that bilberries are remarkable for their anti-oxidant benefits such as macular degeneration prevention, cancer prevention, and their ability to reduce inflammation. Also, the anthocyanosides found in bilberry are said to benefit circulation and reduce the risk of blood clot formation. I think I'll have another slice of Linzer Torte!

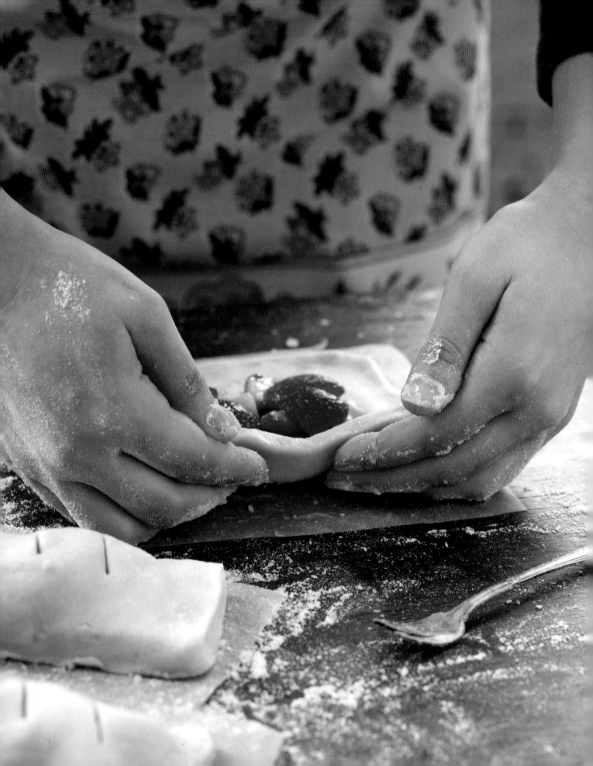

HAND
PIES

◆ ◆ ◆ ◆ ◆

◆ ◆ ◆ ◆ ◆

HAND PIES ARE SO MUCH FUN! Individual pies bursting with flavor add homemade pleasure to any occasion, whether you're having them for dessert around a fancy table, as a snack on a summer picnic, or as an on-the-go breakfast on a chilly morning.

Making these pies can be messy. But just like with anything, with practice, your hand pie finesse will develop. Here are a few tips to aid you in forming a tidy, well-constructed fruit-filled pastry.

HAND PIE TIPS AND TECHNIQUES

SHAPING THE HAND PIES: For aesthetics, I recommend a specific shape for each recipe—a half moon, triangle, or rectangle—although any of those shapes will work fine with any of the fillings. The challenge of shaping the dough is that it's easy to stretch and tear it as you bring it up and over the filling. Alternatively, use the following technique to make a rectangular hand pie that doesn't require folding the dough.

On a well-floured work surface, roll out the dough to a thickness of ⅛ inch. With a sharp knife, cut out 16 rectangles measuring 2½ by 5 inches. Transfer 8 of the rectangles to a baking sheet that's lined with parchment paper or lightly greased. Place the filling in the center of each rectangle. Use a spatula to position the remaining 8 rectangles on top. With a well-floured fork, gently press down around the entire perimeter of the pie to seal the edges.

REPAIRING TEARS IN THE DOUGH: If the dough should tear when you fold it over the filling, don't worry: the hand pie will still turn out fine, and may even be the more charming for it. I have developed the Hand Pie and Turnover Dough recipe (page 21) to allow for extra dough: simply roll and cut out shapes (hearts, leaves, etc.) and place them over any tears.

CREATING FINISHED EDGES: For a crisp look, when sealing the seams of your hand pies, clean up your edges first by using a straightedge such as a knife or razor after the pastry has been folded over the filling. This works well for rectangles and triangles. For half-moon shapes, you can also run your knife very carefully close to the outside edge of the half-moon to make a more precise half circle if you desire a neater appearance. Then crimp the edges gently but firmly with a well-floured fork.

✦ Raspberry Turnovers ✦

Raspberry Turnovers don't last long in my house! I love the way the warm, not-too-sweet filling oozes deliciousness with each bite of tender pastry. When raspberries are in season, I make extra turnovers and freeze them to bake throughout the winter.

‖‖‖‖‖‖‖‖‖‖‖‖‖‖‖‖‖‖‖‖‖‖‖‖‖‖‖‖‖‖‖ **MAKES 8 TURNOVERS** ‖‖‖‖‖‖‖‖‖‖‖‖‖‖‖‖‖‖‖‖‖‖‖‖‖‖‖‖‖‖‖‖‖

EQUIPMENT: 14-by-18-inch rimless baking sheet

1 Hand Pie and Turnover Dough
  (page 21)

½ cup seedless raspberry jam
1 pound fresh raspberries
  (about 2 cups)

‖‖‖

1. Prepare the dough as instructed.

2. Lightly flour your work surface with brown rice flour. Divide the dough into 10 equal balls. Cut eight 7-inch squares of parchment paper and dust them generously with brown rice flour. Roll out 8 of the dough balls into 5-inch-diameter circles on the parchment. (Use the extra dough balls to roll out shapes to cover any tears that occur when you form the pies; see "Shaping the hand pies" and "Repairing tears in the dough," page 89.) Transfer the dough circles on their parchment paper to a rimless baking sheet.

3. Preheat the oven to 375 degrees F.

4. In a small bowl, gently mix the jam and raspberries. Spoon a scant ¼ cup of the filling into the center of each dough circle. Use the parchment paper to gently lift the dough and fold it in half over the filling, creating a half-moon. Form a seal by gently pressing the edges together with a well-floured fork, or crimp the edges with your clean fingers. Using a sharp knife, make 3 small slits in the top of each turnover to allow steam to escape. Freeze the turnovers, uncovered, on the baking sheet for 20 minutes. (The pies can be stored in the freezer at this point to be baked later. Transfer them to an airtight container; they will keep for up to 2 months. Bake them straight from the freezer, on a baking sheet, for 42 minutes.)

5. Bake the turnovers until golden brown, about 30 minutes. Let the pies cool slightly before serving. The baked turnovers will keep for 3 days in the refrigerator; reheat in the microwave or oven.

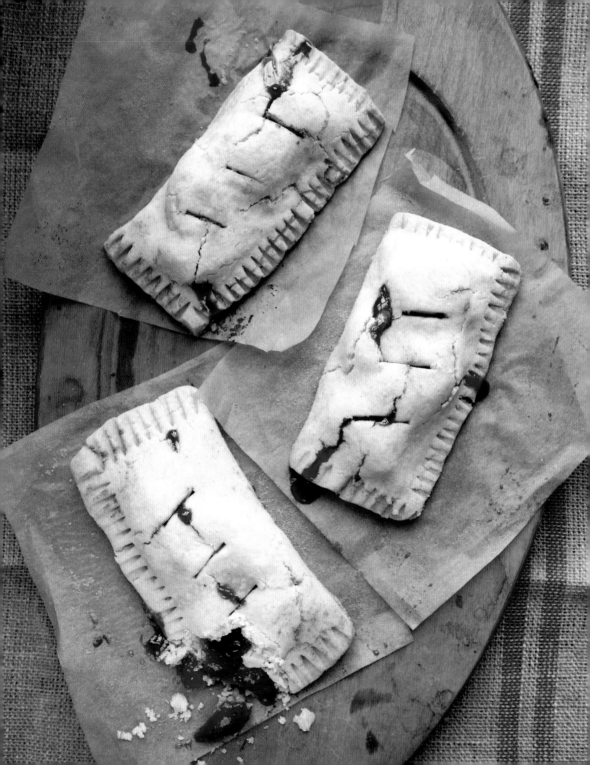

✦ Strawberry Hand Pies ✦

I first made this recipe with my daughter, Lilli, and her friend Noah. Lilli was three and Noah was almost four. While I don't recommend making hand pies with young kids if you're a perfectionist or want them to hold together, we had a ball! These pies require nimble hands and take a bit of artful tenacity, but do involve your family if you want to have a great time and hone those skills together.

‖‖‖‖‖‖‖‖‖‖‖‖‖‖‖‖‖‖‖‖‖‖‖‖‖‖‖‖‖ **MAKES 8 HAND PIES** ‖‖‖‖‖‖‖‖‖‖‖‖‖‖‖‖‖‖‖‖‖‖‖‖‖‖‖‖‖

EQUIPMENT: 14-by-18-inch rimless baking sheet

1 Hand Pie and Turnover Dough
(page 21)

2 pounds fresh strawberries, hulled
and quartered (about 3 cups)

3½ tablespoons evaporated cane juice
or Sucanat

2 tablespoons arrowroot

Sanding sugar or turbinado sugar, for
sprinkling the pies (optional)

‖‖‖

1. Prepare the dough as instructed.

2. In a medium bowl, mix the strawberries, evaporated cane juice, and arrowroot. Let the mixture sit for about 15 minutes while you roll out the dough.

3. Lightly flour your work surface with brown rice flour. Divide the dough into 10 equal balls. Cut eight 7-inch squares of parchment paper and dust them generously with brown rice flour. Roll out 8 of the dough balls into a 5-inch squares on the parchment. (Use the extra dough balls to roll out shapes to cover any tears that occur when you form the pies; see "Shaping the hand pies" and "Repairing tears in the dough," page 89.) Transfer the dough squares on their parchment paper to a rimless baking sheet.

4. Preheat the oven to 425 degrees F.

5. Spoon 2 tablespoons of the filling into the center of each dough square. Use the parchment paper to gently lift the dough and fold it in half over the filling, creating a rectangle. Form a seal by gently pressing the edges together with a well-floured

continued

fork, or crimp the edges with your fingers. Using a sharp knife, make 3 small slits on the top of each hand pie to allow steam to escape. Freeze the pies, uncovered, on the baking sheet for 20 minutes. (The pies can be stored in the freezer at this point to be baked later. Transfer them to an airtight container; they will keep for up to 1 month. Bake them straight from the freezer, on a baking sheet, for 35 minutes.

6. Sprinkle the pies generously with sanding sugar. Bake until golden brown, about 25 minutes, or until golden brown and filling oozes and bubbles. Let the pies cool slightly before serving. The baked pies will keep for 3 days in the refrigerator; reheat in the microwave or oven.

Ever consider growing your own strawberries at home? Strawberries are a delight to grow mainly because they require very little effort. They are also great producers of fruit (just one strawberry plant can produce a quart of berries!), and they are quite generous as a perennial that multiplies each year. Strawberries can be grown out of a pot on a deck, or even a balcony or patio! They will fit nicely in a small or large garden space as long as there is ample sunlight. To get all the nitty-gritty gardening tips to ensure a bountiful harvest, visit StrawberryPlants.org.

✦ Blackberry Hand Pies ✦

In my neighborhood, come August, there are blackberries galore growing on every foot trail, at the end of pedestrian bridges, in backyards, and around the perimeter of soccer fields. The abundance of this scrumptious fruit ensures many blackberry pies in my house.

|||||||||||||||||||||||||||||||||||||||||||| **MAKES 8 HAND PIES** ||||||||||||||||||||||||||||||||||||||||||||

EQUIPMENT: 14-by-18-inch rimless baking sheet

1 Hand Pie and Turnover Dough
   (page 21)

1 pound fresh blackberries (about
   3 cups)

1 tablespoon arrowroot

1 tablespoon brown rice flour

¼ cup packed dark brown sugar

⅛ teaspoon almond extract

Sanding sugar or turbinado sugar, for
   sprinkling the pies (optional)

||||||||||||||||||||||||||||||||||||||||||||||||||||||||||||||||||||||||||||||||||||||||||||||||||||||||||||||||||||||||||||||||||||||||||

1. Prepare the dough as instructed.

2. Lightly flour your work surface with brown rice flour. Divide the dough into 10 equal balls. Cut eight 7-inch squares of parchment paper and dust them generously with brown rice flour. Roll out 8 of the dough balls into 5-inch circles on the parchment. (Use the extra dough balls to roll out shapes to cover any tears that occur when you form the pies; see "Shaping the hand pies" and "Repairing tears in the dough," page 89.) Transfer the dough circles on their parchment paper to a rimless baking sheet.

3. Preheat the oven to 400 degrees F.

4. In a medium bowl, gently combine the blackberries, arrowroot, brown rice flour, brown sugar, and almond extract. Spoon ¼ cup of the filling into the center of each dough circle. Use the parchment paper to gently lift the dough and fold it in half over the filling, creating a half-moon. Form a seal by gently pressing the edges together with a well-floured fork, or crimp the edges with your clean fingers. Using a sharp knife, make 3 small slits in the top of each pie to allow steam to escape. Freeze the

continued

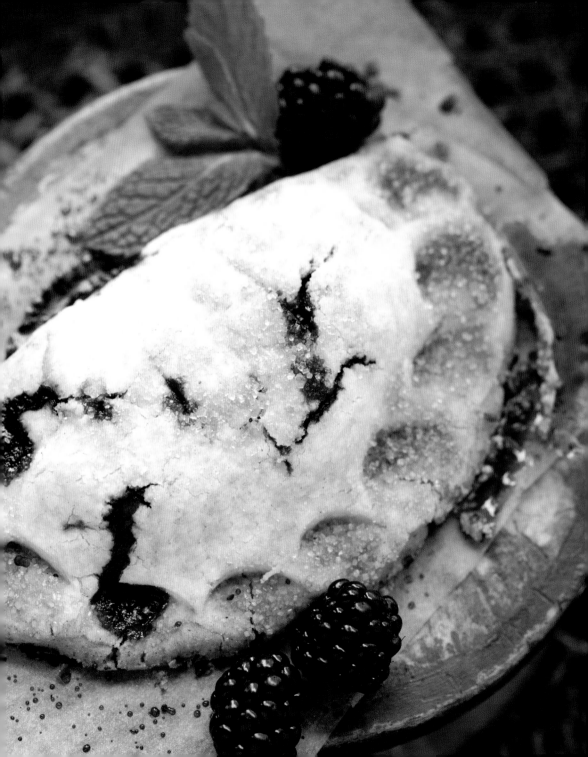

pies, uncovered, on the baking sheet for 20 minutes. (The pies can be stored in the freezer at this point to be baked later. Transfer them to an airtight container; they will keep for up to 2 months. Bake them straight from the freezer for 35 minutes.)

5. Sprinkle the pies generously with sanding sugar. Bake until golden brown, about 25 minutes. Let the pies cool slightly before serving. The baked turnovers will keep for 3 days in the refrigerator; reheat in the microwave or oven.

IT IS SUCH A TREAT TO HAVE BERRIES THROUGHOUT THE WINTER! During berry season, pick to your heart's content with the plan to freeze what you won't be able to enjoy immediately. To freeze blackberries you will need freezer bags, a tray that will fit in your freezer, and a strainer or a colander. Begin by carefully rinsing your berries in cold water with the aid of your strainer or colander. Let the berries drain for about 15 minutes. Spread the dry berries in one layer in a flat tray that will fit in your freezer. Put the berry-lined tray in the freezer until the berries are completely frozen, about 8 hours. Once frozen, transfer the berries to freezer bags. Remove as much air as possible from the bag before sealing them shut to prevent freezer burn. Enjoy your summer-picked berries throughout the winter with porridges, pancakes, and muffins!

✦ Apricot Hand Pies ✦

This recipe calls for dried Turkish apricots, which are then rehydrated. If you haven't used these amazing dried fruits in this way before, you're in for a heavenly and addictive experience. You may even find yourself making the filling more often than the pies. The filling is amazing on toast or mixed into applesauce, yogurt, or porridge.

‖‖‖‖‖‖‖‖‖‖‖‖‖‖‖‖‖‖‖‖‖‖‖‖‖‖‖‖‖‖‖‖‖‖ **MAKES 8 HAND PIES** ‖‖‖‖‖‖‖‖‖‖‖‖‖‖‖‖‖‖‖‖‖‖‖‖‖‖‖‖‖‖‖‖‖‖‖

EQUIPMENT: 14-by-18-inch rimless baking sheet

1 Hand Pie and Turnover Dough
   (page 21)

⅔ pound dried Turkish apricots
   (about 2 cups)

1 tablespoon plus 1 teaspoon
   vanilla extract

½ teaspoon lemon zest

2 tablespoons freshly squeezed
   lemon juice

¼ cup evaporated cane juice

Pinch of salt

Sanding sugar or turbinado sugar, for
   sprinkling the pies (optional)

‖‖‖

1. Prepare the dough as instructed.

2. Place the apricots in a small saucepan and cover with water. Bring the water to a boil, then reduce the heat to a simmer. Cover the pan and let the apricots simmer for 3 hours, until they plump. (Alternatively, you can soak them in a bowl of room-temperature water overnight.) Drain the apricots.

3. In the bowl of a food processor, combine the apricots, vanilla, lemon zest and juice, evaporated cane juice, and salt. Puree until the mixture has a smooth, jam-like consistency.

4. Lightly flour your work surface with brown rice flour. Divide the dough into 10 equal balls. Cut eight 7-inch squares of parchment paper and dust them generously with brown rice flour. Roll out 8 of the dough balls into a 5-inch squares on the parchment. (Use the extra dough balls to roll out shapes to cover any tears that occur when you form the pies; see "Shaping the hand pies" and "Repairing tears in the dough," page 89.) Transfer the dough squares on their parchment paper to a rimless baking sheet.

5. Preheat the oven to 375 degrees F.

6. Spoon ¼ cup of the filling into the center of each dough square. Use the parchment paper to gently lift the dough and carefully fold one corner of the square over the filling to meet the opposite corner, forming a triangle. Form a seal by gently pressing the edges together with a well-floured fork, or crimp the edges with your clean fingers. Using a sharp knife, make 3 small slits in the top of each hand pie to allow steam to escape. Freeze the pies, uncovered, on the baking sheet for 20 minutes. (The pies can be stored in the freezer at this point to be baked later. Transfer them to an airtight container; they will keep for up to 2 months. Bake them straight from the freezer, on a baking sheet, for 42 minutes.)

7. Sprinkle the pies generously with sanding sugar. Bake until golden brown, about 35 minutes. Let the pies cool slightly before serving. The baked pies will keep for 3 days in the refrigerator; reheat in the microwave or oven.

✦ Chaussons aux Pommes ✦

An autumn treat that always gratifies! Serve these for breakfast, with afternoon tea, or as an evening dessert à la mode. My daughter and I like to make these hand pies throughout the apple season. We delight in the different flavors as one apple variety goes out of season and another emerges.

|||||||||||||||||||||||||||||||||||||||||||||||| **MAKES 8 PIES** ||||||||||||||||||||||||||||||||||||||||||||||||||

EQUIPMENT: 14-by-18-inch rimless baking sheet

1 Hand Pie and Turnover Dough
    (page 21)

¾ pound tart apples, such as Pink
    Lady or Granny Smith

¾ pound sweet apples, such as Cameo,
    Ambrosia, or Red Delicious

¼ cup water

2 tablespoons evaporated cane juice

½ teaspoon lemon zest

1 teaspoon freshly squeezed
    lemon juice

|||||||||||||||||||||||||||||||||||||||||||||||||||||||||||||||||||||||||||||||||||||||||||||||||||||||||||||||||||||||||||

1. Peel and core the apples and cut them into 1-inch-thick slices. In a medium saucepan, combine the apple slices, water, evaporated cane juice, and lemon zest and juice. Bring to a boil, then reduce the heat to a simmer and cover the pan. Simmer for 15 minutes, stirring occasionally. Remove the pan from the heat, and with a fork, slightly mash the apples. Let the filling cool completely.

2. Meanwhile, prepare the dough as instructed.

3. Lightly flour your work surface with brown rice flour. Divide the dough into 10 equal balls. Cut eight 7-inch squares of parchment paper and dust them generously with brown rice flour. Roll out 8 of the dough balls into a 5-inch squares on the parchment. (Use the extra dough balls to roll out shapes to cover any tears that occur when you form the pies; see "Shaping the hand pies" and "Repairing tears in the dough," page 89.) Transfer the dough squares on their parchment paper to a rimless baking sheet.

4. Preheat the oven to 400 degrees F.

5. Spoon 2 tablespoons of the filling into the center of each dough square. Use the parchment paper to gently lift the dough and carefully fold one corner of the square over the filling to meet the opposite corner, forming a triangle. Form a seal by gently pressing the edges together with a well-floured fork, or crimp the edges with your clean fingers. Using a sharp knife, make 3 small slits in the top of each hand pie to allow steam to escape. Freeze the pies, uncovered, on the baking sheet for 20 minutes. (The pies can be stored in the freezer at this point to be baked later. Transfer them to an airtight container; they will keep for up to 2 months. Bake them straight from the freezer, on a baking sheet, for 42 minutes.)

6. Bake the hand pies for 15 minutes, then reduce the oven temperature to 350 degrees F. Bake for an additional 15 minutes, or until golden. Let the pies cool slightly before serving. The baked pies will keep for 3 days in the refrigerator; reheat in the microwave or oven.

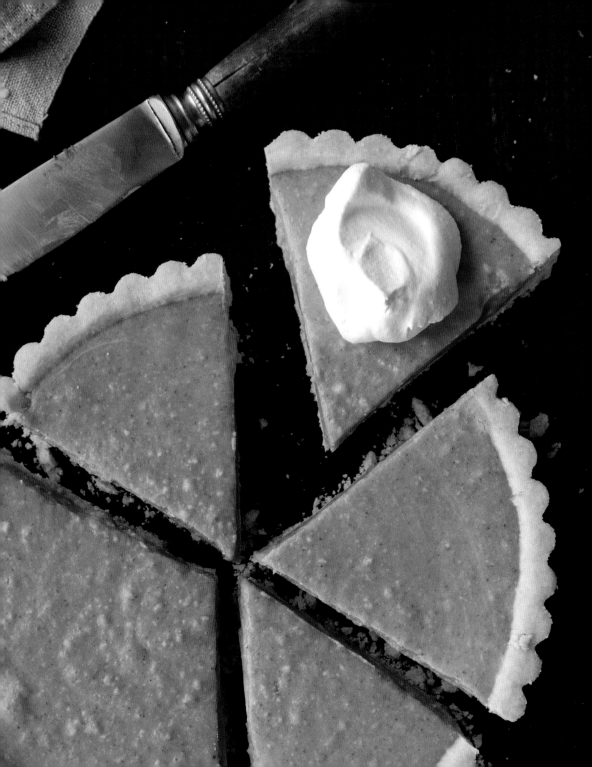

CREAM
PIES

◆ ◆ ◆ ◆ ◆

◆ ◆ ◆ ◆ ◆

THESE FABULOUS CREAM PIES are smooth, silky, fulfilling, and light all at once. Savor each creamy mouthful, as I'm sure they won't last long! In the springtime, minty Grasshopper Pie (page 109) satisfies when summer fruits haven't yet arrived in markets. In the summer, berry cream pies (pages 110, 111) are refreshing and bright. Come fall and winter, Chocolate Cream Pie (page 114) and Pumpkin Chiffon Pie (page 113) are full-bodied and truly gratifying. A great variety of crusts (especially the press-in nut crusts) pair heavenly with the fillings in this chapter.

The inspiration for the luscious filling base of these rich pies comes from Isa Chandra Moskowitz and Terry Hope Romero, who authored the famous *Vegan Pie in the Sky*. Although my recipes are quite different, I was very much influenced by their brilliant idea of combining cashews, coconut milk, and agar.

Note that you'll have to plan ahead when making the pies in this chapter: all require prebaking and cooling the crust at least one and a half hours and up to one day in advance, as well as allowing at least two hours to soak the cashews and four hours for the filling to chill and set in your refrigerator. While all this makes for a lengthy stretch of time before the pie is ready, the steps are easy and each one goes rather quickly.

I like to begin making my cream pies in the morning. At 8 a.m., I set the cashews to soak and then begin making the crust. By 10 a.m., the crust is baked and cooled, and I begin making the cream filling. By 10:30 a.m., the pie is chilling and setting up in my fridge, and as early as 2:30 p.m. I can sneak a slice! If you're in a rush the day of, though, the crust can easily be made the day before, the cashews can be put out to soak very early in the morning, and the filling can be made just before you leave for work in the morning.

Cream Pie Tips and Techniques

SOAKING THE CASHEWS: All of the recipes in this chapter use softened cashews as a filling base. Soak them for at least two hours in a bowl filled with 2 cups cold tap water (ideally filtered). The longer you soak the cashews, the creamier your filling with be; however, don't soak them longer than eight hours, as they'll become rather slimy. If you're pressed for time, using unsoaked cashews or soaking them for less than two hours will still produce a great pie; it will just be a bit less creamy.

TIMING THE CRUST: Prepare and prebake your crust as instructed in the specific crust recipes, and let it cool for about one and a half hours before making your filling. Each filling comes together quickly, and once it's ready, you'll want to immediately pour it into your cooled crust and pop it in the fridge to set.

MAKING THE FILLING: All of the recipes in this chapter call for simmering water, maple syrup, and agar flakes together for five minutes; be sure to stir these ingredients every minute or so to prevent them from burning.

SHOPPING FOR COCONUT MILK: Be sure to use whole, rather than light, coconut milk because the filling is not creamy and rich enough otherwise.

✦ Banana Cream Pie ✦

This was the first cream pie recipe I developed. I found it so extraordinarily delicious, I had to refrain from creating a book solely focused on cream pies! It's superb as it is, but you can also play around with it in a number of ways. For example, garnish the pie with dark chocolate shavings or curls or sprinkle it with toasted slivered almonds.

||||||||||||||||||||||||||||||||||||||||||| **MAKES ONE 9-INCH PIE** |||||||||||||||||||||||||||||||||||||||||||

EQUIPMENT: 9-inch pie pan or 8-inch springform pan

1 Ginger Pecan Press-In Crust (page 28), Almond Press-In Crust (page 26), Chocolate Almond Press-In Crust (page 27), or Dark Chocolate Pecan Press-In Crust (page 30). Or use a Single Pastry Crust (page 9), baked for 40 minutes at 350 degrees F

FOR THE FILLING:

½ cup raw cashews, soaked in water for 2 to 8 hours

3 bananas, divided

One 13-ounce can whole coconut milk

1 tablespoon vanilla extract

Juice of 1 medium lemon

¼ cup water

2 teaspoons agar flakes

½ cup maple syrup

3 tablespoons coconut oil

||||||||||||||||||||||||||||||||||||||||||||||||||||||||||||||||||||||||||||||||||||||||||||||||||||||||||||||||||||

1. Prepare the crust as instructed.

2. Drain the cashews. Place them in a blender or the bowl of a food processor along with 2 of the bananas, coconut milk, vanilla, and lemon juice. Process thoroughly until very creamy and smooth. Leave the mixture in the blender.

3. In a small saucepan, combine the water, agar, and maple syrup. Bring the mixture to a boil, then reduce the heat to a simmer. Simmer for 5 minutes, stirring occasionally, then remove the pan from the heat and stir in the coconut oil. Add this mixture to the banana mixture in the blender and process until emulsified.

4. Slice the remaining banana into ½-inch-thick rounds and arrange them over the crust. Pour the filling over the sliced bananas. Refrigerate the pie and let it set for 4 hours before serving.

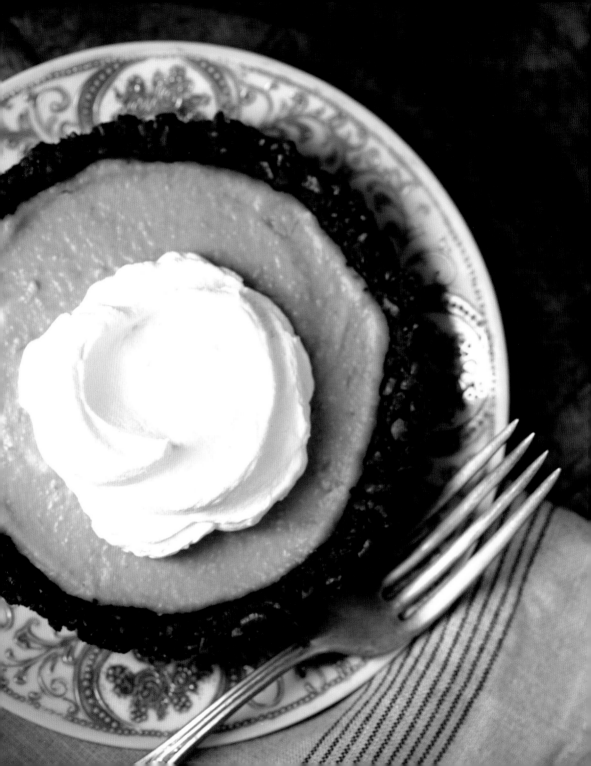

✦ Grasshopper Pie ✦

Although this is a chilled dessert, you may be surprised to find your cheeks warming from the generous amount of crème de menthe in the filling. The addition of avocado makes each bite exquisitely silky. The contrast of the pale green filling with the dark brown chocolate garnish is most eye-catching.

|||||||||||||||||||||||||||||||||||||||||||||||| **MAKES ONE 8-INCH PIE** ||||||||||||||||||||||||||||||||||||||||||||||||||

EQUIPMENT: 8-inch springform pan

1 Dark Chocolate Pecan Press-In Crust (page 30) or Chocolate Almond Press-In Crust (page 27)

¾ cup raw cashews, soaked in water for 2 to 8 hours

1½ avocados

One 13-ounce can whole coconut milk

⅓ cup green crème de menthe

¼ cup water

2 teaspoons agar flakes

½ cup maple syrup

3 tablespoons coconut oil

Dark chocolate shavings or curls, for garnish

||||||||||||||||||||||||||||||||||||||||||||||||||||||||||||||||||||||||||||||||||||||||||||||||||||||||||||||||||||||||||||||

1. Prepare the crust as instructed.

2. Drain the cashews. Place them in a blender or the bowl of a food processor along with the avocados, coconut milk, and crème de menthe. Process thoroughly until very creamy and smooth. Leave the mixture in the blender.

3. In a small saucepan, combine the water, agar, and maple syrup. Bring the mixture to a boil, then reduce the heat to a simmer. Simmer for 5 minutes, stirring occasionally, then remove the pan from the heat and stir in the coconut oil.

4. Add this mixture to the avocado mixture in the blender and process until smooth and creamy.

5. Pour the filling into the crust. Place in the freezer for 40 minutes before serving. Refrigerate the pie and let it set for 4 hours before serving. Garnish with dark chocolate shavings.

⋅ Strawberry Cream Pie ⋅

This pie's texture is somewhere between a mousse and a cheesecake. Fresh pureed strawberries give it a bright flavor and festive pink color. I particularly enjoy this pie with a Ginger Pecan Press-In Crust (page 28).

|||||||||||||||||||||||||||||||||||||| **MAKES ONE 8-INCH PIE** ||||||||||||||||||||||||||||||||||||||

EQUIPMENT: 8-inch springform pan

1 Almond Press-In Crust (page 26), Ginger Pecan Press-In Crust (page 28), Chocolate Almond Press-In Crust (page 27), or Dark Chocolate Pecan Press-In Crust (page 30)

½ cup raw cashews, soaked for 2 to 8 hours

One 13-ounce can whole coconut milk

2 medium bananas

1 pound fresh strawberries, hulled (about 2 cups), plus 5 or 6 strawberries, sliced, for garnish (optional)

1 tablespoon vanilla extract

¼ cup water

3 teaspoons agar flakes

¾ cup maple syrup

3 tablespoons coconut oil

Fresh mint leaves, for garnish (optional)

Dark chocolate curls or shavings, for garnish (optional)

||||||||||||||||||||||||||||||||||||||||||||||||||||||||||||||||||||||||||||||||||||||||||||

1. Prepare the crust as instructed.

2. Drain the cashews. Place them in a blender or the bowl of a food processor along with the coconut milk, bananas, strawberries, and vanilla. Process thoroughly until very creamy and smooth. Leave the mixture in the blender.

3. In a small saucepan, combine the water, agar, and maple syrup. Bring the mixture to a boil, then reduce the heat to a simmer. Simmer for 5 minutes, stirring occasionally, then remove the pan from the heat and stir in the coconut oil. Add this mixture to the strawberry mixture in the blender and process until smooth and creamy.

4. Pour the filling into the crust. Refrigerate the pie and let it set for 4 hours before serving. Place in the freezer for 40 minutes before serving. Line the perimeter of the pie with sliced strawberries, and arrange mint leaves in pairs or trios on top or garnish with dark chocolate shavings.

✦ Blueberry Cream Pie ✦

This pie is vibrant with fresh blueberries blended into the creamy filling, a kick from the ginger in the crust, and a modest amount of sweetener. I love to garnish it with sprigs of fresh mint.

|||||||||||||||||||||||||||||||||||||| **MAKES ONE 8-INCH PIE** ||||||||||||||||||||||||||||||||||||||

EQUIPMENT: 8-inch springform pan

1 Ginger Pecan Press-In Crust
  (page 28)

½ cup raw cashews, soaked in water
  for 2 to 8 hours

1 medium banana

One 13-ounce can whole coconut milk

8 ounces fresh blueberries
  (about 2 cups)

1 tablespoon vanilla extract

Juice of 1 medium lemon

¼ cup water

1 tablespoon agar flakes

½ cup maple syrup

3 tablespoons coconut oil

1. Prepare the crust as instructed.

2. Drain the cashews. Place them in a blender or the bowl of a food processor along with the banana, coconut milk, blueberries, vanilla, and lemon juice. Process thoroughly until very creamy and smooth. Leave the mixture in the blender.

3. In a small saucepan, combine the water, agar, and maple syrup. Bring the mixture to a boil, then reduce the heat to a simmer. Simmer for 5 minutes, stirring occasionally, then remove the pan from the heat and stir in the coconut oil. Add this mixture to the blueberry mixture in the blender and process until well combined and smooth.

4. Pour the filling into the crust. Refrigerate the pie and let it set for 4 hours. Place in the freezer for 40 minutes before serving.

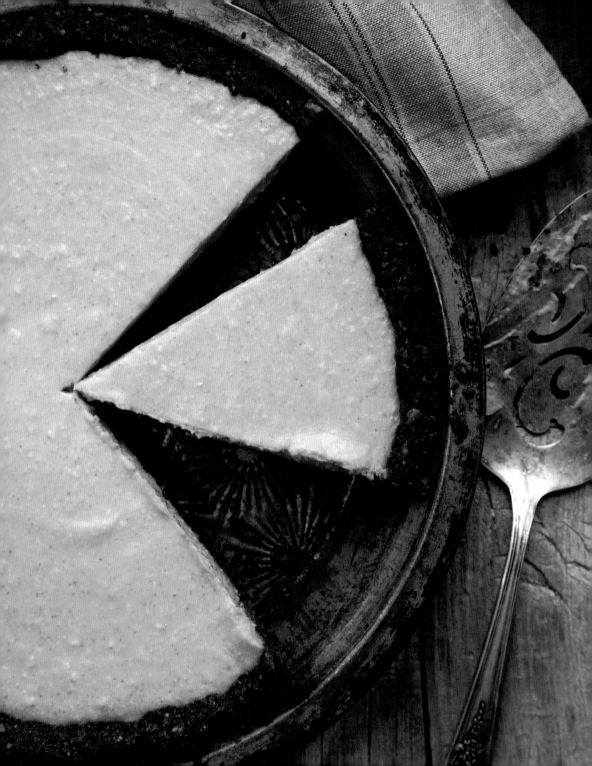

✦ Pumpkin Chiffon Pie ✦

Delectable Pumpkin Chiffon Pie is light and perfectly balanced with spice. I predict you'll be eating it not just for Thanksgiving but throughout the fall and winter seasons. Make it in a springform pan with one of the lovely press-in nut crusts or make the pastry crust in a pie pan and place decorative pastry leaves on top. (Please note, should you choose to make the Single Pastry Crust (page 9), you can use the extra dough after fitting your pie pan to make the leaves. The leaves will take 15 minutes to bake on a separate sheet pan. They are beautiful as a garnish, after the pie has chilled and set.)

|||||||||||||||||||||||||||||||||||||||||||| **MAKES ONE 9-INCH PIE** ||||||||||||||||||||||||||||||||||||||||||||

EQUIPMENT: 9-inch springform pan or pie pan

1 Almond Press-In Crust (page 26), Hazelnut Pastry Crust (page 18), or Ginger Pecan Press-In Crust (page 28). Or use a Single Pastry Crust (page 9), baked for 40 minutes at 350 degrees F

½ cup raw cashews, soaked in water for 2 to 8 hours

One 15-ounce can pumpkin puree

One 13-ounce can whole coconut milk

1 tablespoon vanilla extract

1 teaspoon ground cinnamon

¼ teaspoon ground cloves

¼ teaspoon ground nutmeg

¼ teaspoon ground ginger

¼ cup water

2 teaspoons agar flakes

½ cup maple syrup

3 tablespoons coconut oil

||||||||||||||||||||||||||||||||||||||||||||||||||||||||||||||||||||||||||||||||||||||||||||||||||||||||||||||||||||||||||||||||||

1. Prepare the crust as instructed.

2. Drain the cashews. Place them in a blender or the bowl of a food processor along with the pumpkin, coconut milk, vanilla, cinnamon, cloves, nutmeg, and ginger. Process thoroughly until very creamy and smooth. Leave the mixture in the blender.

3. In a small saucepan, combine the water, agar, and maple syrup. Bring the mixture to a boil, then reduce the heat to a simmer. Simmer for 5 minutes, stirring occasionally, then remove the pan from the heat and stir in the coconut oil. Add the mixture to the pumpkin mixture in the blender and process until smooth and creamy.

4. Pour the filling into the crust. Refrigerate to let the pie set for 4 hours before serving.

✦ Chocolate Cream Pie ✦

This silky-smooth pie is unbearably good. The chocolate filling, while rich, is not as intense as that of the Chocolate Prune Tart (page 82) or Chocolate Espresso Tart (page 81), but instead tastes more like milk chocolate. I particularly enjoy this pie with a Dark Chocolate Pecan Press-In Crust (page 30). Garnish it with dark chocolate shavings or curls, or strawberries dipped in dark chocolate next to a sprig of fresh mint.

||||||||||||||||||||||||||||||||||||||| **MAKES ONE 9-INCH PIE** |||||||||||||||||||||||||||||||||||||||||

EQUIPMENT: 9-inch pie pan or 8-inch springform pa

1 Almond Press-In Crust (page 26), Ginger Pecan Press-In Crust (page 28), Chocolate Almond Press-In Crust (page 27), or Dark Chocolate Pecan Press-In Crust (page 30), made in an 8-inch springform pan. Or use a Single Pastry Crust (page 9), made in a 9-inch pie pan and baked for 40 minutes at 350 degrees F

½ cup raw cashews, soaked in water for 2 to 8 hours

One 13-ounce can whole coconut milk

1 tablespoon vanilla extract

½ cup water

2 teaspoons agar flakes

¼ cup Sucanat

¼ cup maple syrup

1 tablespoon coconut oil

3½ ounces unsweetened dark chocolate

||||||||||||||||||||||||||||||||||||||||||||||||||||||||||||||||||||||||||||||||||||||||||||||||||||||||||||||||||||||||

1. Prepare the crust as instructed.

2. Drain the cashews. Place them in a blender or the bowl of a food processor along with coconut milk and vanilla. Process thoroughly until very creamy and smooth. Leave the mixture in the blender.

3. In a small saucepan, combine the water, agar, Sucanat, and maple syrup. Bring the mixture to a boil, then reduce the heat to a simmer. Simmer for 5 minutes, stirring occasionally, then remove the pan from the heat and stir in the coconut oil. Add this mixture to the cashew mixture in the blender.

4. Melt the chocolate over low heat in a double boiler or a stainless steel bowl set over a small saucepan filled with about 2 inches of gently simmering water. (The bowl should not touch the water.) Add the melted chocolate to the mixture in the blender and process until smooth and creamy.

5. Pour the filling into the crust. Refrigerate the pie and let it set for 4 hours.

DARK CHOCOLATE ISN'T JUST PLEASING BECAUSE IT TASTES OH SO decadent. In fact, dark chocolate actually releases amorous endorphins (called Phenylethylamine) in our brains shortly after we eat some. These chocolate-induced endorphins are the same endorphins released when we are falling in love!

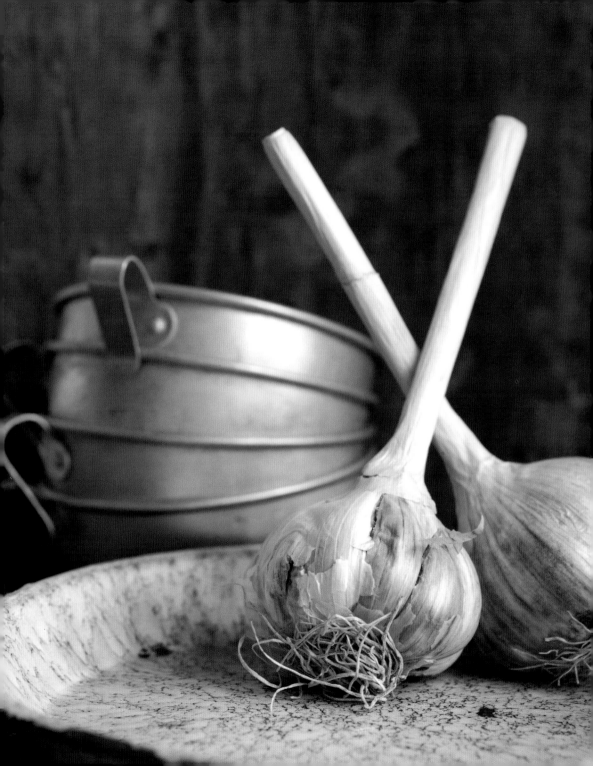

SAVORY
PIES

◆ ◆ ◆ ◆ ◆

Spring Risotto Torte with Asparagus
and Porcini Mushrooms 120

Layered Eggplant Tarts with
Pistachio Crusts 123

Savory Provençal Tart 125

White Bean and Broccoli Rabe Tart 127

Tamale Pie 130

Asian Potpie 133

Curried Parsnip Pie 134

◆ ◆ ◆ ◆ ◆

A SAVORY PIE IS A FESTIVE PRESENCE on a lunch or dinner table. These full-flavored entrees are welcoming and evoke curiosity—what's inside that delicious-looking pie wafting such pleasing smells? Savory pies, while growing in popularity, are still not as common as sweet pies where I live. Often sweets have the upper hand when it comes to luring us in, but you're about to find out that savory pies deserve a lot more of our attention. In fact, instead of choosing savory over sweet, or sweet over savory, make both for your next gathering!

Each recipe in this chapter is quite different from the next in ingredients and flavor, and several include their own special crust specific to the filling that accompanies it. Finally, each recipe is abundant with vegetables; do pay attention to sauté times when making your fillings to achieve the ultimate flavor and texture.

✦ Spring Risotto Torte with Asparagus and Porcini Mushrooms ✦

This creamy torte offers tasty asparagus spears and bits of succulent porcini mushrooms with each mouthful. Don't be afraid of making the risotto: the process can be both exciting and relaxing. Taking care that the rice absorbs the wine and stock before adding the next ladleful ensures a wonderful texture that's well worth your attention. The torte needs to be refrigerated overnight, so plan accordingly.

|||||||||||||||||||||||||||||||||||| **MAKES ONE 8-INCH TORTE** ||||||||||||||||||||||||||||||||||||

EQUIPMENT: 8-inch springform pan, fine-mesh sieve

2 ounces dried porcini mushrooms

4 cups boiling water

1 pound asparagus

¼ cup extra-virgin olive oil, plus more for oiling the pan

½ cup gluten-free bread crumbs

2 medium onions, diced

3 cloves garlic, minced

1¾ cups arborio rice, rinsed to remove extra starch

1½ cups white wine

Pinch of salt

Freshly ground pepper

½ cup finely chopped Italian parsley, for garnish

|||||||||||||||||||||||||||||||||||||||||||||||||||||||||||||||||||||||||||||||||||||||||||||||||||||||

1. Soak the porcinis in the boiling water for 1 hour.

2. While the mushrooms soak, trim off the tough ends of the asparagus and chop the stalks into 1-inch pieces. Lightly steam them in a steamer basket over boiling water for 5 minutes. Set aside.

3. Lightly brush an 8-inch springform pan with olive oil and coat with the bread crumbs, shaking out the excess. Set aside.

4. Gently lift the mushrooms out of the water, being careful not to stir up any grit that may have settled at the bottom of the dish. Squeeze the mushrooms dry, coarsely chop them, and set them aside. Strain the mushroom soaking liquid through a fine-mesh sieve lined with cheesecloth or a paper towel. In a small

saucepan, bring the liquid, which is your mushroom stock, to a simmer, maintaining that simmer throughout the risotto-making process.

5. In a large soup pot, heat the oil over medium-low heat. Add the onions and garlic and sauté for 10 minutes. Add the mushrooms and cook for another 2 minutes. Add the rice and cook, stirring, until it becomes lightly translucent, about 7 minutes. Increase the heat to medium-high and add the wine and salt. Cook, stirring continuously, until the wine is almost completely absorbed, about 15 minutes. Add a ladleful of mushroom stock and cook until it's completely absorbed, stirring constantly. Continue this process until all the mushroom stock is absorbed into the rice. Taste a piece of rice; it should be tender yet firm to the bite. Remove the risotto from the heat and stir in the asparagus. Season to taste with pepper and additional salt.

6. Spoon the risotto into the prepared pan and smooth it with a spatula. Let the risotto cool completely before placing it in the refrigerator overnight.

7. Preheat the oven to 400 degrees F.

8. Bake the torte for 30 minutes, or until heated through. Carefully unmold the torte onto a serving platter. Slice it into wedges and garnish each wedge with parsley.

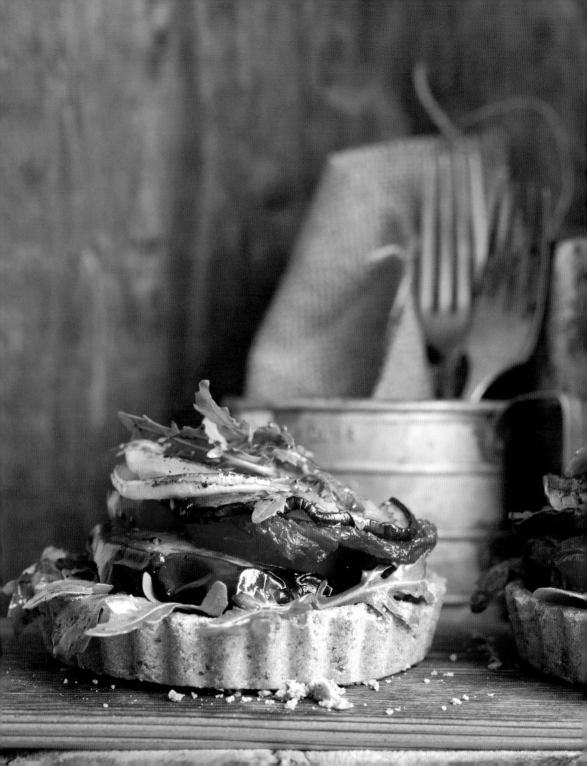

✦ Layered Eggplant Tarts with Pistachio Crusts ✦

Visually, these individual layered tarts are like sculptural towers. The pistachio crust is mildly sweet and salty. The simple yet vibrant layers of roasted eggplant and peppers, caramelized onion, sun-dried tomatoes, and fresh arugula interact with gusto. Enjoy these tarts freshly made for a dinner party, or make them earlier in the morning and serve them at room temperature for a luncheon.

|||||||||||||||||||||||||||||||||||||||||| **MAKES 6 SMALL TARTS** ||||||||||||||||||||||||||||||||||||||||||

EQUIPMENT: Six 3-inch tart pans

FOR THE CRUST:
2 cups salted shelled pistachios
¼ cup canola oil
½ cup teff flour
2 tablespoons maple syrup
¼ cup water

FOR THE FILLING:
2 medium eggplants, sliced into
    ¼-inch-thick rounds (about 6 slices
    per eggplant)
½ cup olive oil, divided

3 tablespoons balsamic vinegar
½ teaspoon salt
2 medium onions, thinly sliced into
    half-moons
3 cups arugula
1 teaspoon salt
1 cup jarred roasted red peppers
⅔ cup oil-packed sun-dried tomatoes,
    drained
1 tablespoon fresh oregano leaves,
    for garnish

||||||||||||||||||||||||||||||||||||||||||||||||||||||||||||||||||||||||||||||||||||||||||||||||||||||||||||||||||||||||||||||||

1. To make the crust, preheat the oven to 350 degrees F.

2. Combine the crust ingredients in the bowl of a food processor and process just until the dough begins to hold together but still has a lot of texture from the pistachios. Divide the dough into 6 equal portions and press each into a 3-inch tart pan. Place the tart pans on a baking sheet, and place the sheet on the middle rack of the oven. Bake the crusts for 22 minutes.

continued

3. Remove the crusts from the oven and set aside to cool. Increase the oven temperature to 400 degrees F.

4. To make the filling, place the eggplant rounds on a baking sheet lined with parchment paper and drizzle them with 6 tablespoons of the olive oil and the balsamic vinegar, then sprinkle with the salt. Bake for 40 minutes, or until they're cooked through and slightly crisped.

5. In a medium skillet, heat the remaining 2 tablespoons oil over medium-low heat. Add the onions and sauté for 15 minutes, or until just beginning to brown. Add the arugula and stir briefly just to wilt it. Set aside.

6. Remove the tart crusts from their pans and place them on a serving platter or directly on individual plates. To assemble the tarts, divide half of the sautéed onions and arugula among the 6 tart shells, reserving the other half. Next, place an eggplant slice on top of each tart. Divide the red peppers among the tarts. Divide half of the sun-dried tomatoes among the tart shells, reserving the other half. Place another slice of eggplant on each tart and divide the remaining portion of the onions and arugula among the tarts, followed by the remaining portion of sun-dried tomatoes. Garnish each tart with a sprinkle of fresh oregano. Serve warm or at room temperature.

✦ Savory Provençal Tart ✦

This tart comes together quickly, although one would assume otherwise when admiring it on the dining table. It's full of Mediterranean goodness: tomatoes, rich olives, sautéed onions and garlic, pine nuts, capers, and Provençal herbs. You can prepare the crust as early as the morning prior to filling and serving it. I like this tart with a tossed green salad and crusty baguette—perhaps one from my Gluten-Free and Vegan Bread *book!*

|||||||||||||||||||||||||||||||||||| **MAKES ONE 9-INCH TART** ||||||||||||||||||||||||||||||||||||||||

EQUIPMENT: 9-inch fluted round tart pan

FOR THE CRUST:

1 cup brown rice flour

⅓ cup potato starch

¼ cup teff flour

½ teaspoon salt

1 teaspoon herbs de Provence

½ cup palm fruit oil or coconut oil

¼ cup toasted pine nuts

FOR THE FILLING:

3 tablespoons olive oil

2 large onions, finely chopped

3 cloves garlic, chopped

One 15-ounce can diced tomatoes

1 teaspoon evaporated cane juice

Leaves from 1 sprig thyme

⅔ cup pitted kalamata olives, chopped

3 tablespoons capers

Salt and freshly ground pepper

Chopped Italian parsley, for garnish

||||||||||||||||||||||||||||||||||||||||||||||||||||||||||||||||||||||||||||||||||||||||||||||||||||||

1. To make the crust, preheat the oven to 375 degrees F.

2. Combine the brown rice flour, potato starch, teff flour, salt, herbs de Provence, and palm fruit oil in the bowl of a food processor and process just until the dough begins to hold together. Add the pine nuts and pulse briefly to combine. Press the dough into a 9-inch fluted round tart pan, level off the dough with the pan sides, and pierce it all over with a fork. Place the pan, uncovered, in the freezer for 20 minutes, then transfer it directly to the oven and bake for 25 minutes. Remove from the oven and set aside to cool for 1 hour before filling.

continued

3. To make the filling, in a large skillet, heat the oil over medium heat. Add the onions and garlic and sauté for 15 minutes, or until just beginning to brown. Add the tomatoes, evaporated cane juice, and thyme leaves and sauté for another 15 minutes. Remove the pan from the heat and stir in the olives and capers. Season with salt and pepper to taste.

4. To assemble the tart, spoon the filling into the crust and smooth the top. Sprinkle the parsley over the tart and serve it warm or at room temperature.

⬩ White Bean and Broccoli Rabe Tart ⬩

This savory tart is rich in Italian splendor. The oil pastry makes a slightly nutty and scrumptious crust, surrounding a robust filling of garlic, rosemary, pungent greens, and creamy beans. The pastry may feel oily and perhaps looser than you may be expecting: use your hands to press the dough into place, and it will bake up handsomely.

IIIIIIIIIIIIIIIIIIIIIIIIIIIIIIIIIIIIIII **MAKES ONE 10-INCH TART** IIIIIIIIIIIIIIIIIIIIIIIIIIIIIIIIIIIIIII

EQUIPMENT: 10-inch tart pan with a removable bottom

FOR THE CRUST:

1 cup brown rice flour

⅓ cup medium-grind cornmeal

¼ cup tapioca flour

½ teaspoon salt

½ cup canola oil

½ cup chopped toasted walnuts

FOR THE FILLING:

1 medium bunch broccoli rabe (also known as rapini), tough stems removed

2 tablespoons olive oil

3 garlic cloves, minced

2 cups cooked white lima beans or other white beans, or two 15.5-ounce cans, rinsed and drained

1 teaspoon minced fresh rosemary

Salt and freshly ground pepper

¼ cup chopped toasted walnuts

IIIIIIIIIIIIIIIIIIIIIIIIIIIIIIIIIIIIIIIIIIIIIIIIIIIIIIIIIIIIIIIIIIIIIIIIIIIIIIIIIIIIIIIIIIIIIIIIIIIIIIIIIIIIIIIIIIIIIIIIIIIIIIIIIIIIIIIIIIIIIIIIIIIII

1. To make the crust, preheat the oven to 375 degrees F.

2. Combine the brown rice flour, cornmeal, tapioca flour, salt, and oil in the bowl of a food processor and process just until the dough holds together. Add the walnuts and pulse briefly to combine. Press the dough into a 10-inch tart pan. Bake for 35 minutes.

3. To make the filling, bring a large pot of salted water to a boil. Cook the broccoli rabe until tender, about 5 minutes. Drain it in a colander, then run it under cold water. Coarsely chop and set aside.

continued

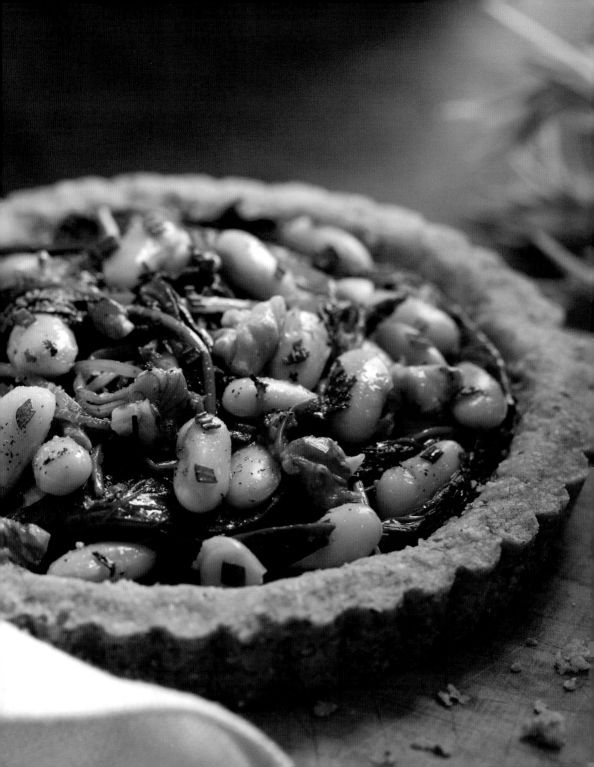

4. In a large skillet, heat the oil over medium heat. Add the garlic and sauté for just under 1 minute. Stir in the beans and rosemary, then add the broccoli rabe and season with salt and pepper to taste. Cook until everything is heated through, about 7 minutes. Pour the filling into the crust, top with the walnuts, and serve immediately.

BROCCOLI AND BROCCOLI RABE HAVE ALMOST THE SAME NAME, but they are quite different. Broccoli is mild and sweet tasting, while broccoli rabe is deliciously bitter and powerfully strong. Broccoli is closely related to cauliflower, while broccoli rabe is a relative of the turnip! Both vegetables were brought over to the states by Italian farmers around the same time in the early 1900s, however broccoli rabe is still a lesser known exotic vegetable. If you haven't tried broccoli rabe already, I'm confident that you are about to have your taste buds awakened by a vegetable rich with Italian splendor.

✦ Tamale Pie ✦

This Latin-spiced pie fills a 10-inch springform pan right up to the brim. A hearty serving of layered polenta, black beans, peppers, and spiced vegetables goes a long way with a generous dollop of guacamole and a bit of fresh salsa. Leftovers carry over deliciously, and the pie can easily be rewarmed for about 20 minutes in a hot oven or toaster oven with a covering of foil. You can prepare and assemble it the day before serving.

|||||||||||||||||||||||||||||||||||||||| **MAKES ONE 10-INCH PIE** ||||||||||||||||||||||||||||||||||||||||||||

EQUIPMENT: 10-inch springform pan

2 tablespoons olive oil

1 medium onion, finely chopped

2 teaspoons chili powder

1 small zucchini, chopped

2 medium tomatoes, chopped

1 orange bell pepper, stemmed, seeded, and diced

2 cups chopped butternut squash, or one 10-ounce frozen package

1½ cups cooked black beans, or one 15-ounce can, rinsed and drained

2 teaspoons salt, divided

2 tablespoons fresh oregano leaves, divided

4 cups water

1¾ cups polenta

||||||||||||||||||||||||||||||||||||||||||||||||||||||||||||||||||||||||||||||||||||||||||||||||||||||||||||||||||

1. Preheat the oven to 350 degrees F.

2. In a large skillet, heat the oil over medium-low heat. Add the onions and sauté until they're just beginning to become transparent, about 5 minutes. Add the chili powder and zucchini and sauté until the zucchini begins to brown slightly, about 7 minutes. Add the tomatoes, bell pepper, squash, beans, 1 teaspoon of the salt, and 1 tablespoon of the oregano. Mix well and reduce the heat to low. Let the mixture cook while you prepare the polenta.

3. In a large saucepan, bring the water, polenta, and remaining 1 teaspoon salt to a boil, then reduce the heat to a simmer and cook for 7 minutes, stirring continuously. Remove the polenta from the heat.

4. Divide the polenta into 3 equal portions. Pour one-third into a 10-inch spring-form pan and use a spatula to spread the polenta over the entire bottom. Top this with half of the bean and vegetable filling, then the next third of the polenta, followed by the second half of the filling, and finally, the last third of the polenta. Sprinkle the remaining 1 tablespoon oregano over the top, cover the pan with aluminum foil, and bake on the lower rack of the oven for 1 hour. Serve immediately.

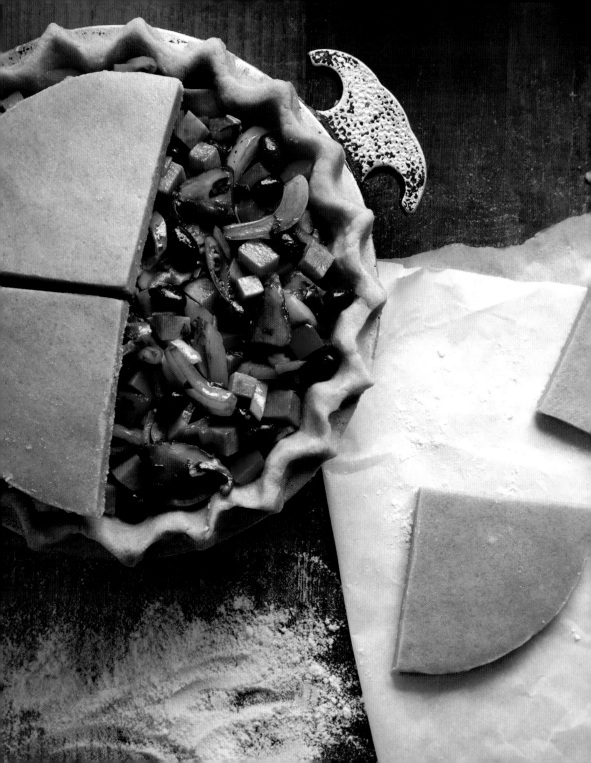

✦ Asian Potpie ✦

I find this satiating, warming, and yummy potpie to be especially nourishing on cold evenings. The portobello mushrooms contribute a hearty texture; the sweet potato adds sweetness, of course; and the sugar snap peas and bok choy are fresh and brightening. Being a lover of greens, I like to serve this potpie with a side of simply steamed kale drizzled with olive or sesame oil and sprinkled with sea salt and sesame seeds.

‖‖‖‖‖‖‖‖‖‖‖‖‖‖‖‖‖‖‖‖‖‖‖‖‖‖‖ **MAKES ONE 9-INCH POTPIE** ‖‖‖‖‖‖‖‖‖‖‖‖‖‖‖‖‖‖‖‖‖‖‖‖‖‖‖‖‖

EQUIPMENT: 9-inch pie pan

1 Darker Double Crust (page 14) with a wedge top crust

2 tablespoons canola oil

1 medium onion, chopped

3 cloves garlic

½ teaspoon dried summer savory

2 tablespoons tamari

2 large portobello mushrooms, cut into 1-inch pieces

1 medium sweet potato, peeled and diced

1 medium red bell pepper, stemmed, seeded, and diced

One 15-ounce can black beans, rinsed and drained

1 cup sugar snap peas

3 heads baby bok choy, chopped

‖‖

1. Prepare the crust as instructed.

2. Preheat the oven to 375 degrees F. Place a baking stone or aluminum foil–lined baking sheet on the middle rack of the oven.

3. In a large skillet, heat the oil over medium heat. Add the onions and garlic and sauté until the onions begin to soften and become transparent, about 10 minutes. Add the summer savory, tamari, mushrooms, sweet potato, and bell pepper. Let the vegetables simmer for about 15 minutes before adding the black beans, sugar snap peas, and bok choy. Mix well, then spoon the filling into the prepared bottom crust. Spread the filling out evenly, then arrange the wedge top crust.

4. Place the pie on the baking stone or sheet. Bake for 1 hour. Serve piping hot.

✦ Curried Parsnip Pie ✦

This pie is comforting in the fall and winter months when parsnips are at their best. Rich curried coconut milk envelops thick slices of sweet parsnips, colorful vegetables, and chickpeas, all bound by a wholesome and tender crust. The dough is delicate, so it's a bit more challenging to work with than other doughs in this book, but it's so flavorful that it's worth the extra effort. Enjoy this dish with steamed greens or a crisp salad.

|||||||||||||||||||||||||||||||||||| **MAKES ONE 10-INCH PIE** ||||||||||||||||||||||||||||||||||||

EQUIPMENT: 10-inch pie pan

FOR THE FILLING:

2 tablespoons canola oil

1 medium onion, thinly sliced into half-moons

2 teaspoons coriander seeds

2 teaspoons mustard seeds

1 tablespoon curry powder

14 ounces green beans, cut into 1-inch pieces (about 1 cup)

2 medium parsnips, sliced into disks about ¼-inch thick

2 medium tomatoes, cut into wedges

1 sweet potato, sliced into half-moons about ¼ inch thick

1½ cups cooked chickpeas, or one 15-ounce can

One 13-ounce can coconut milk

1 teaspoon salt

FOR THE CRUST:

2 cups quinoa flour

1 cup teff flour

1 teaspoon salt

½ cup canola oil

¼ cup plus 2 tablespoons water

1 tablespoon maple syrup

½ cup flax meal

3 tablespoons coconut oil

||||||||||||||||||||||||||||||||||||||||||||||||||||||||||||||||||||||||||||||||||||||||||||||||||||||||

1. To make the filling, in a large skillet, heat the oil over medium heat. Add the onions and sauté until they soften and become transparent, about 5 minutes. Add the coriander seeds, mustard seeds, and curry powder and continue sautéing until the seeds begin to pop, about 3 minutes. Add the green beans, parsnips, tomatoes, sweet potato, chickpeas, coconut milk, and salt and simmer for 12 minutes, or until the vegetables begin to soften. Remove the pan from the heat and set aside.

2. Preheat the oven to 350 degrees F.

3. To make the crust, place the flours and salt in the bowl of a food processor and process just until combined. Add the canola oil, ¼ cup of the water, maple syrup, flax meal, and coconut oil and process just until the dough holds together.

4. On a surface well dusted with brown rice flour, divide the dough in half. Press one half into a 10-inch pie pan and crimp the edges. Pour the filling into the crust. Return remaining dough to the food processor and pulse the remaining 2 tablespoons water into the dough.

5. On a surface well dusted with brown rice flour, roll the dough out to about a ¼ inch thickness. Using a well-floured glass, cut out circles, or with a well-floured cookie cutter or freehand, cut out leaves or other shapes. Arrange the cutouts over the filling so that they overlap around the perimeter of the pie, leaving the center of the filling exposed.

6. Place the pie on the baking stone or sheet. Bake for 1½ hours, or until the filling is bubbling up and the crust is golden. Serve immediately.

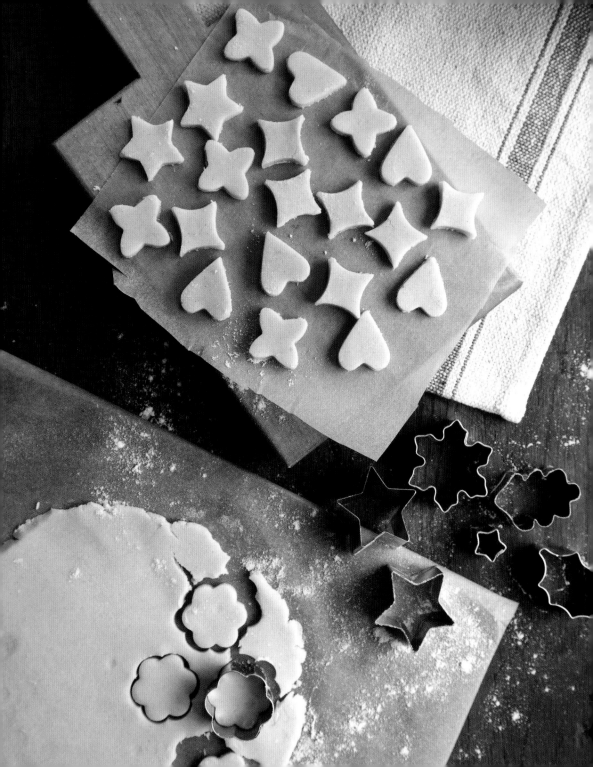

INDEX

About the Author

JENNIFER KATZINGER and her father first opened the doors of the Flying Apron Bakery in 2002, recognizing the value in organic, gluten-free, vegan, and sustainable whole foods years in advance of what has become a rapidly expanding industry. After growing the bakery from a tiny take-out window in Seattle's University District to a spacious and lovely café in the city's Fremont neighborhood, Jennifer sold the bakery in 2010, and it continues to thrive.

After selling the bakery, Jennifer pursued her two greatest passions: being a mother, and continuing to develop delicious and healthy recipes. She is delighted to bring you her fourth cookbook! Knowing that gluten-free and vegan pastry is quite a rare find, she is thrilled to share these scrumptious new pie recipes.

Jennifer earned a BA in English Literature from the University of Washington, and pursued a Master's in Industrial Design from the Pratt Institute in Brooklyn, New York. She lives in Seattle with her husband, Joseph; their daughter, Lillian; and their dog, Neve. They enjoy taking long walks through the beautiful parks of the Pacific Northwest and creating delicious, nurturing food together.

ABOUT THE PHOTOGRAPHER

CHARITY BURGGRAAF is a photographer whose "rustic meets modern" vision of food has been recognized in publications nationally and internationally. She has a great passion for her subject matter, and the community it brings together. She lives in Seattle.

ABOUT THE FOOD STYLIST

JULIE HOPPER learned to style food in the pressure-filled studios of Chelsea and Hell's Kitchen in New York City. She's styled for major national food magazines including *Bon Appetit*, *Cooking Light*, and *O, The Oprah Magazine*. Julie's playful yet precise style is now at home in the Pacific Northwest, resulting in many enticing cookbook collaborations.

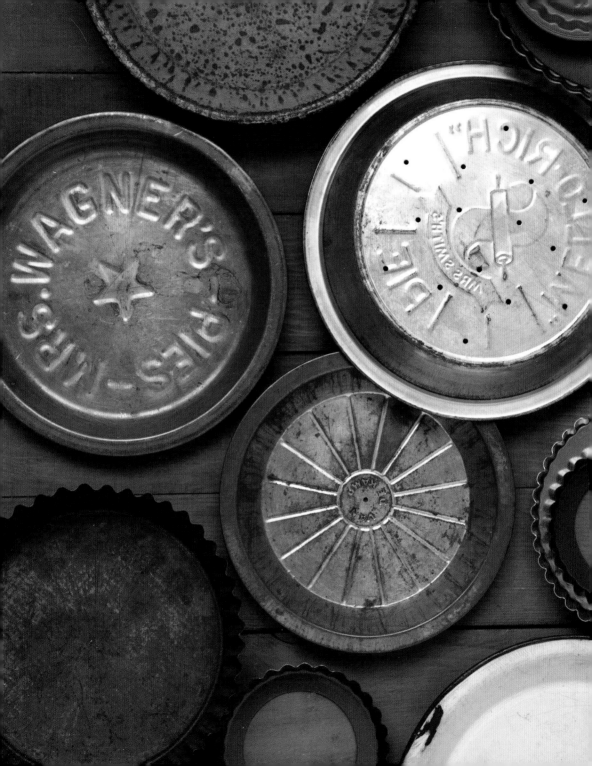